*How many calamities
does it take to make a baby?*

# Introduction

THE JOURNEY TO having a child should be a simple one, shouldn't it? A man meets a woman, or a woman meets a man. They date, get married, have a child, and live happily ever after.

But what if that's not the case?

What happens when a woman meets a woman or a man meets a man?

The world is ever-changing, and these types of relationships are now more recognised. My story is about two women on the quest to have a child and then, ultimately, a woman as a singleton becoming a mother.

Taking you through the ups, the downs, the in-between bits and everything else, I'll be as honest as possible and hopefully make you smile.

I also hope that I can give you hope on your journey to becoming a parent through IVF (in vitro fertilisation*).

But before we turn the page and begin, be sure to have a large mug of tea, a full biscuit tin, and a tissue or two ready.

Oh, and one more thing: where I have put an *, there is a handy glossary at the end of the book, which explains in more detail what the word or term means, along with some helpful references.

# Chapter 1
## They Didn't Teach Me That At School!

I WANTED TO use this chapter to point out a few important things. Sounds very corporate, doesn't it? But believe me, it isn't really.

Firstly, a woman and a woman can have a child, but not in the conventional way. I attended those school personal and social education lessons and now understand how birds and bees can make babies. But I also know that unless there is miracle, it is impossible to have a child as a same-sex couple. Believe me when I say I tried that.

Secondly, when I'm at the hospital for any other issue except for being in labour, when you ask if I'm pregnant and I say no, that it's a firm no (even more so if my girlfriend is standing right next to me)! I think I would remember if I'd been through an IVF, intrauterine insemination (IUI*), or some similar procedure.

Sometimes life can throw you those 'wonderful' curved balls, as I discovered, of polycystic ovary syndrome and endometriosis along the way.

My journey also takes in weight loss. There are three words I can use to sum this up. It is hard! Short and sweet.

An IVF journey can be confusing, complicated, sad, frustrating, make you angry, and create numerous other emotions. Many times along the way, you will want to throw in the towel and question why it is so hard. Then, you take a deep breath, pull your socks up, and get on with it.

One of my most important beliefs is that I am not a number on a spreadsheet that somebody can enter into a statistical report or some pawn that a doctor can move into checkmate on a chessboard. Is it even possible for pawns to be in checkmate?

No, I am a person with feelings, a heart and a soul. I hurt just like anyone else and deserve the utmost respect during such a difficult time. Sadly, numerous people often neglected this on my particular road.

And probably the most crucial point for you is that I don't sugarcoat anything. Over the years,

I have learned not to do that. I'm a big believer in telling it as it is. There is no point in beating around the bush, as that leads to confusion, heartache, and not knowing all the facts.

There you have it—just a few simple things to get us started on the road.

# Chapter 2
## Let's Start At The Very Beginning

THAT'S A VERY good place to start.

Let's step into that time machine and go back to when I was 11 years old. This was when I got my first period—a rite of passage in any woman's life. We think, 'Oh, that's my period', when we have a few days of uncomfortableness, a bit of blood, and then it disappears until the next month.

That is the dream scenario, isn't it? Some women have this, and I'd say they are very lucky. Some of us have 'issues' which can last a year or years. They can leave us questioning whether womanhood is the right direction for us and wanting to rip out our ovaries and womb to stop the pain that rips through our bodies every month, and finally debating whether white clothes are a good choice during your tsunami period when you have to attend a formal work function.

I was always a bit of an early bloomer. My breasts developed early, hormones raged, and I had a very spotty face, so it was no surprise that my period appeared early on in my life. I did that British thing of just getting on with it and didn't really feel the need to discuss it with friends. My mum was a family planning doctor at the time, so if there were any questions regarding the situation, she could answer them.

Maybe that was the right thing to do, or perhaps it wasn't. Who knows! What I will say is that it needs to be on your terms.

If you're a chatterbox and over a glass of wine on a Friday night, feel the need to discuss the inner most details of your menstrual cycle with anyone who will listen, then fill your boots and have no shame or embarrassment about it.

If you're like me and prefer the quieter side of things, that's OK, too.

Or you could turn all your thoughts into a book! It's entirely up to you.

Over the years, I have had trouble with my periods: late ones, full-on heavy ones, hormones on the rampage and general ickiness. Nothing was investigated, examined or diagnosed until, as a 20-year-old, I presented to my GP with 'period issues'. My period had disappeared and failed to return for months at a time. It had gone on for several months before getting to the GP stage.

At last, I was sent for some blood tests to see if we could find the answer to the question or if this was the way my period was going to operate.

After I received a phone call calling me into the surgery to discuss my blood results, I found myself in my GP reception area waiting for my name to be called. I knew that GPs would only call you in if there was a problem, so clearly they had found something in my blood and maybe had an explanation as to why my periods were being a pain in the you-know-what.

I was told by the GP I had PCOS (polycystic ovary syndrome*), along with the devastating news that the likelihood of me becoming a mother would be tough to non-existent at that time.

Now, for someone who knew from a very early age that she wanted to be a mum, this was far from 'excellent news'.

I watched as my dream of becoming a mother vanished quickly. I remember being devastated by this news, and I avoided places children would be. Even walking past a playground on the way to work or holding someone else's child while they dug the latest toy out of their bag was too much for me to cope with.

At the time, there wasn't much help to deal with these emotions, so I buried them deep inside and then carried on as if nothing had happened.

I should point out that this was in 2004 when there was not much science behind these issues, and everything was still being 'researched'.

Throughout my twenties, I still had issues with my period and with weight around my middle. I didn't think much of it. My periods were sore and were so heavy that I always carried two spare changes of clothes. I had to have two or three pairs of the same trousers and a full pack of sanitary pads with me during my time of the month. Heavy periods are just horrendous. You're constantly on edge when out and about, terrified that you'll have 'an accident'. On top of that, you have incredibly sore ovaries and back pain. I always used to say that they were playing tennis or that a big band was tightening around my middle. The lower back was not much fun either when it decided to get in on the act as well.

I was prescribed the contraceptive pill and went with two different varieties at the time. For me, I didn't feel I got on with the medication terribly well, though. I felt that my emotions, which were all over the place at the best of times, ended up even more chaotic. I was angry, sad, happy, hyperactive, and confused, all in the space of a few minutes.

It was awful, and this was all on the quest to grow into being a woman. Sometimes, I wish you could pick your own gender or choose whether to have ovaries and the associated pain, discomfort, mood swings, headaches, and nausea that go with being a woman. It may have been easier earlier on to make these choices, and if I had not wanted children so badly, I would have asked for a refund from Mother Nature or whoever is in charge of these things.

When I reached my thirties, things started to change. On one occasion, I approached the GP with a lot of pain in my groin lymph nodes. I had previously had some trouble when I had had an infection in them, which resulted in me being in hospital and on strong antibiotics. I thought I was having a recurrence of this, so I popped along to the GP, who did a whole bunch of tests 'down there'. The question came about my cycle, and I answered, 'Painful and heavy.' The doctor asked whether I had tried the coil.

"No, what is that?" I asked.

After an explanation and a clear STI (sexually transmitted diseases) test, I was booked in to have one fitted.

After several failed attempts by a nurse to perform this procedure at the local GP practice, it had become so incredibly painful and traumatic that the nurse had to stop before she caused me any further distress, and my coil was thankfully fitted in the local hospital under a general anaesthetic a few weeks later, which was a great relief.

All I can remember about that time is the pain while the coil got things under control. I was sore;

my ovaries hurt, my back ached, and I felt like my middle was being squashed in a vice. To top it all off, I had a continuous discharge of old blood.

I was told to persevere with the journey as it was just the coil getting things under control. My goodness, I was all for taking it out after a week or so, as the pain was awful.

After around six weeks, things calmed down, and I had the coil for just under five years. It made a massive difference in slowing things down and helping my hormones and emotions get back in check.

I went from flying off the handle and being angry to having long periods of being calm and focused. The period didn't stop completely, but it was enough to have a regular cycle with minimal pain. If asked about my periods over those five years, I had a good answer about when they may appear. I thought this was a great achievement as I feel it is the right of a woman to know this. I mean, there are those little apps you can get on your phone now with period calendars, which I thought were cool, but I could never have one as I never knew when or if the thing would appear.

# Chapter 3
## Disaster Strikes

WHILE LIVING IN London, I had been training for the Richmond Park Duathlon*. I like to give myself fitness challenges, and this is the biggest one I would tackle. I did a lot of cycling when I lived in London, completed numerous charity rides ranging from 10 to 50 miles, raised money for charity along the way, and had loads of fun. Who else would like climbing a hill on an overnight ride at mile 59 of a 60-mile challenge?

It was demanding and fun, made me feel alive, and I was doing a good thing raising money for various charities.

I entered to do the half duathlon event, which meant I would do a 5km run, 20km cycle, and another 5km run. It was going to be a challenge because me and running didn't see eye-to-eye at times (unless it was running for the bus, so I wasn't late for work).

I spent months cycling, running, doing strength and conditioning work in the gym, stretching, preparing and eating the right foods. I was in the best shape that I could be in for taking part.

Then disaster struck!

I woke up on the Wednesday morning and didn't feel right. I thought maybe I had a bug or something, or perhaps I'd over-trained. With the level I had been doing, it could have been the reason and the one I hoped for. I didn't eat breakfast that morning but pulled myself together for my final training run. When I say run, I was walking more than anything. At the time, I was with my girlfriend, who had run ahead of me to get her last run in. By the time she got back to where I was hobbling along, I was almost doubled over.

We thought it best to get to the GP to see what was going on, and maybe with a day's rest, everything would be fine. At the GP's, my temperature was through the roof, along with my blood pressure and pulse. The prodding and poking around my abdomen left me in agony, and I was quickly dispatched to A&E with suspected appendicitis.

At the emergency department, I had a variety of tests and scans to see if they could pinpoint what was going on. I even had a nurse ask if I was pregnant. I, of course, said no.

"Are you sure?" she asked.

"Yes, I'm sure, considering my other half is a woman. I'm aware of the birds and the bees and even I know there is a vital ingredient missing between two women."

Luckily, the consultant arrived during this conversation and said a pregnancy test was unnecessary. It will always baffle me when women are asked this question and are not taken at face value with their answers. Anyway, I was booked in for an overnight stay in the hospital so they could monitor me and see how I was the following morning.

Once on the ward during one of the checks, the nurse asked me how much exercise I was getting. I explained that I was training for the duathlon, and it soon became more of a question about how much rest I was getting rather than the exercise. At this point, over training was ruled out as the contributing factor.

I seemed to be in one of those big wards on my own, so it was a tad lonely at times, but someone wheeled in a TV to help me beat the loneliness and boredom. Now, I don't know if it's my imagination, but it seems that every time I get sick or end up in the hospital, there seems to be a programme about baking. When you're bordering on hallucinations from the drugs, it puts a whole new spin on the cakes being awesome—the colours, in particular, lead to a lot of hilarity.

The next day, Thursday, the doctor came around and did some more prodding on my abdomen. He was concerned that I seemed to be getting worse rather than better and booked me in for emergency exploratory surgery later that morning. I came round from surgery convinced I would be fit enough to run, cycle and participate in the Sunday duathlon. But as the surgeon had completed keyhole surgery through my belly button and straight through my stomach muscles, I was going nowhere. I was devastated. Despite all my hard work, dedication and commitment to training, I was to go no further.

Post-surgery, the surgeon came to say that my appendix looked normal, but they had taken it out as a precaution. He also said that I had had a cyst on my ovary, which had burst and flooded my abdomen with disgustingness, hence all the symptoms. Nothing at this point was said about endometriosis. I would have thought he would now have an idea of what was happening, but apparently not. I suspected he was a general medical surgeon rather than the gynaecology team, which would make sense.

The following morning, I was discharged to recover at home. I admit that bending in the middle due to the incision was troublesome. Even the basics of going from sitting to standing or standing to sitting was tricky. I couldn't even do the simple tasks of getting dressed, and putting my socks and shoes on was nearly impossible. I had to come up with fun ways to do things.

A few days later I turned up with my girlfriend at the duathlon start line. Well, she was still booked to do it, and I was insistent that she go ahead without me. I had to watch from the side lines. I admit that it was an incredibly hard day for me watching all those people run and cycle, but supporting a family member helps take the sting out of things a bit.

During my recovery, I walked everywhere I could. I started with a few steps and built it up. From there, I began to do gentle abdominal work and cycling. Progressing further, I graduated to bigger weights and longer cycle rides. Being an exercise rehab personal trainer did help enormously as well. In a few months, I had recovered enough to go back to long-distance cycle rides, but I didn't go back to running at this point. I hung up my running shoes for now and concentrated on what I knew best: cycling.

# Chapter 4
## The London IVF Clinic

AFTER I HAD recovered fully from my surgery, my girlfriend and I started talking about families. I had always known I wanted children, and I felt that as I was in a secure and loving relationship, it was time to start exploring options to get the process going. Being the youngest of us, I would go forwards with whatever was thrown at us to have a child.

Living in London, I thought approaching my local GP was a good place to start. We were booked for an appointment at our local hospital a few months after the original meeting.

All I will say about that is it was a short timescale, as in England at that time, getting IVF was more of a paid activity than doing it on the NHS. It was deemed, even though we were in a same-sex partnership, we would not be permitted to use the NHS option as that was reserved for people who had tried and failed to do it the conventional way.

I translated the 'conventional way' to mean 'heterosexual couple or straight'. Now, with the times fast-changing and IUI, IVF, surrogacy, using one partner's egg into the womb of another woman, and everything else in between, I was confused as to why a woman and a woman couple were not permitted access to this NHS service.

Our only options were to move boroughs in London and try again or to stump up the cash. I did the calculations and discovered we would need something in the region of £7k for one round. Making it work with London's prices, rents, and salaries would not be feasible. It would have taken several years to raise that sum of cash, and that was for one cycle only.

Someone mentioned that we could try a crowd-funding exercise, but it didn't seem to sit right with me, so I never tried it. I was aware that people do it, and I wish them good luck, but it was not the right way forwards for me.

We put the whole idea on the back burner to see where we would be in a year or so and how best to make the dream of becoming parents work. In the meantime, I kept my exercise in check, my nutrition on point and attended information evenings on adoption, fostering, surrogacy and everything in between.

I went to a breakfast event in East London one day specifically for LGBTQ+ (Lesbian, Gay, Bisexual, Transgender, Queer or Questioning) couples, but it didn't really shed any further light on the subject, and I continued in the research phase of proceedings for many a month to come. I often wondered why it wasn't simple and what I needed to do to make it easier. A lot of reading was involved, and I tried to stay as positive as possible.

After my emergency surgery, I didn't appear to have any further issues with my ovaries for another year or so. The coil stayed in and did its job, and I got on with life.

My girlfriend and I decided it was time to move out of London, and Scotland was our destination. I'm originally from Glasgow, so it made sense to head back to this neck of the woods. I wanted my family close by for when the time came to welcome a little one into the world, and in London, my friends seemed to be dotted North, South, East and West, and it could take up to an hour for them to get to me if there was an emergency. Where I now live, I only have a 10 to 15-minute car ride to my parents' house. It's also just an hour's drive to the Loch Lomond National Park hills, but that's another story.

I changed jobs, then changed jobs again, and got a new home to rent, where I finally had my own car parking spot and a wee garden. Anyone with a car who has lived in London without a parking space will understand how important this is! Generally, I was just getting on with life.

My next 'issue' was a lot milder than the emergency surgery I had had in London. This time, I went straight to the GP with similar symptoms, bypassed A&E, and ended up at the local hospital's gynaecology department. A scan the following morning confirmed that I had another small burst ovarian cyst. There was no major intervention this time, thankfully just bed rest, painkillers and some monitoring. A few days later, after that magical cocktail of rest, I was fit and well again to continue life.

The subject came up again about IVF as I began to realise that any ovarian cyst could lead to much wider consequences and potential removal of vital parts of my reproductive organs. It was time to see what Scotland could offer for IVF.

# Chapter 5

## Would I get IVF in Scotland?

GOING THE USUAL route into IVF in Scotland started with a visit to the GP when I explained that my girlfriend and I were looking to start a family and asked what we needed to do.

After a few anxious months of waiting, a letter arrived to say we could go to our local hospital to see a nurse in the fertility department.

Off I popped. There was the mandatory weigh-in, height check, blood pressure taken and blood tests before going home that day with a follow-up with the consultant a couple of weeks later.

At this appointment, I received the first blow on our journey towards having a child. The long and short of our consultation was that I was too overweight to be put on the IVF wait list. I weighed in at 106 kilograms, which put me overweight by about 18 kilograms. My BMI was calculated at 35.8, which put me in the obese category.

Now, to get into the Scotland IVF programme, you need a BMI of 29.9 as the bare minimum, or it is a no-go.

In comparison, 18kg is similar to 18 bags of 1kg of sugar, so it was a lot of weight.

Anyway, back to the consultation, which I think was poorly handled. I don't know what it is about some of these consultants who feel they can act high and mighty. They seem to think they can dictate to everyone. But that was pretty much what happened. This was the second time in my life that I was told that having children would be tricky. This time it was that I was too overweight to go down the 'having children road'. The consultant pretty much said to go away, lose weight and then when you think you are there, come back to us. That was it. There was no other advice, education or help. Nothing!

Now, I was in a very fortunate position as a personal trainer and knew the basics of weight loss. I was going to try my hardest to get my weight down. What I didn't know at this point was how much of a topsy-turvey weight loss journey I would go on with ovarian issues and hormones.

It took me weeks to recover from visiting that consultant. It felt very much like a factory. Yes, you're in. Nope, not you. Yes, you can go, but no, not you. It was like a conveyor belt of potential mothers, all with their own characteristics. It was horrible and a situation I still feel needs to be better equipped and to have more understanding medical professionals.

There really was no alternative. I got myself under control and began my weight loss plan. This journey would take me around 18 months to complete and would become a roller-coaster of emotions, gym time, nutrition, nutritionists and research galore.

Let me sum up my weight loss journey for you in two words:

F*cking hard!!!

There you go. It's as simple as that. Any weight loss journey has different levels of difficulty. I guess it depends on how your body handles the change. Everything for me changed, and today, as I write this chapter, I see that there are several elements in my life that have changed so much. My old nutrition and exercise are now non-existent, never to be seen again. I altered my entire life during the process. I believe in a lifestyle change rather than a quick weight-loss fix, and I guess I experienced it that way. I like to do what I preach.

Sometimes, people say that a weight loss journey is not a race and that taking part is just as important. That is the case. If you want a quick fix, it is just that, quick! Sure, you will get the results over a week to fit into that little black dress for a night out, but then come the following week, when you start eating your old diet, hey presto, your weight will reappear. Weight loss, to me, is, and always has been, a lifestyle change. It takes time. Things need to change. You need a good goal at the end of it and tonnes and tonnes of determination.

During the process, I changed my meals, mealtimes, meal prep, food groups (more on that later!), portion sizes, my exercise programme, my life, my body, my family, and so on. I wish there was a magic way of doing it as I could have avoided a lot of the heartache, tears, sweat and confusion, but seeing as I am not a multi-millionaire with a magic potion, there isn't. A successful weight loss journey takes a lot of hard work, dedication, and changes.

I think during a weight loss journey, it comes down to two things:

## 1) How badly do you want it?

What is your ultimate goal, and is that goal strong enough to pull you forwards when the going gets tough and you want to throw in the towel?

## 2) Are you ready to work hard?

How much effort are you willing to put into achieving your goal, and do you have enough determination to succeed?

At the end of the day, that is the magic formula (well, in my book, anyway, as I was the one to experience first-hand all of what I have just said).

The bottom line for me during the weight loss was if I wanted to get on to the IVF waiting list and be in with a chance of trying to get pregnant, then the weight had to come off.

If I wasn't bothered, then the weight could stay, and there would be no entry to 'Mum Land' for me. Once you get such a powerful goal behind you, it will help massively in the whole weight loss journey.

That second question goes hand in hand with the first one. If you have a powerful goal, then the hard work is easier. You have something to aim towards. It will still be challenging, but it is slightly more manageable if you have a toolbox full of tools to help you and the ability to adapt to changes.

When I started my weight loss journey, I admit I started the wrong way. I didn't change my nutrition. I exercised more, but nothing else. In a month, I had lost less than half a kilo. It was a pathetic return for my hard work in the gym and not a great start.

The following month, I changed my nutrition and continued exercising. I lost three kilos.

I can hear you all shouting at me as you read this, "If you're a personal trainer, why didn't you see that?"

That is a valid question, and the short answer is that I didn't put two and two together to come up with the conclusion. I spent my days discussing nutrition with people but rarely turned the question around to myself. It was one of those situations where I was too close to see the obvious. It suddenly made a lot of sense once I had time to think about it. The results showed that changing the nutrition and carrying on with the exercise levels was the magic formula.

From my Personal Trainer school days, I learned that 70% of a weight loss journey was about nutrition and the other 30% involved exercise. You can see straight away where the main objective lies.

Weighing scales! Those innocent-looking little scales can cause a lot of problems when you are on a weight loss journey.

One thing I encountered repeatedly when asked to stand on these was that unless you were using the same brand, every set of scales is different and can have varied readings. I think the greatest variance in scales was a half to two kilograms. Now, in the grand scheme of things, this was a LOT! It could be the difference between getting into an IVF service or not. The hospital scales and my own scales were case in point here.

The IVF criteria says your BMI must be a maximum of 29.9, but they leave it there. Surely, there must be a different system, one that works for everyone and, in my personal opinion, fairer than the current one. Now, I'm not saying this just because I didn't get my way, but I feel the IVF criteria were then, and are still, out of date. I will explain further in the next chapter why I think this and use examples for better understanding. I also managed at one point to rant to someone in about an hour with 22 new points I would like to add or change about the current system.

I am open to anyone who oversees the IVF system in Scotland to meet me for coffee (maybe without cake) so I can explain. I understand that in Scotland, we are fortunate to get a free go at the procedure on the NHS, but I still believe the criteria should be reviewed.

Please note, in England, we were turned down from moving forwards with IVF as we were not in a borough which supported two women getting pregnant unless there was a known medical issue for why we couldn't. Being a same-sex couple was not a sufficient reason. We were told we either had to move to a different borough or pay for it.

I am all for putting some money towards the IVF procedure, but £7K a pop seems ludicrous.

# Chapter 6
## A Bad Diet Will Always Win

THE BIGGEST LESSON I learned is that you cannot outrun a bad diet. You can exercise as much as you like, but if the nutrition is not there to back up the exercise, you will likely be going one step forwards and two steps backwards. Yes, it will give you more exercise, but still not get you to lose weight

As I mentioned earlier, the weight loss ratio is 70% for nutrition and 30% for exercise. At the start of my weight loss journey, I would say that I was hovering around 80% in exercise and 20% in nutrition. No wonder I didn't lose anything during that first week. You need a massive nutritional overhaul to make weight loss work.

I have completed some research to prove my point a bit more (I love a bit of research). Here's what I found during my trawl through many papers, social media, websites, documentaries and books.

I'll keep it brief:

## Sugary Drinks

A sugary soft drink will take 26 minutes of walking or 13 minutes of running to burn off. It may take five minutes to drink, but is it worth it?

## Blueberry Muffins

If you go to your favourite coffee house and eat a blueberry muffin at 265 calories, it will take 48 minutes of walking or 25 minutes of running to burn off. If you add in a grande white chocolate mocha, the calories keep going up, and there is even more time needed to burn it off.

## Crisps

My final example is crisps (a personal favourite, I have to admit). If you eat a small packet of crisps at 171 calories, you need 31 minutes of walking or 16 minutes of running to burn it off.

As you can see, you can't outrun a bad diet, and it all comes down to what I have said; the magical formula of 70% nutrition and 30% exercise.

Once I'd realised that I needed nutrition to help me with weight loss, I began to make some big changes. These were:

**Food**

I replaced my usual sugary cereal with porridge or yoghurt (low fat, low sugar and no fun!) with fruit and a sprinkle of nuts or healthier cereal (corn or bran flakes).

Lunch that had previously been a sandwich, crisps and a yoghurt, changed to a fried egg wrap with fruit, or something else egg-related, or a salad with ham.

My huge dinner potions were now a much smaller affair, and I only had treats on a rare occasion. For dinner, I had wholemeal pasta, chicken and rice, a massive salad, baked potato with beans, tacos, naked hamburgers and so on.

If I needed a sweet treat, it was an apple, banana, strawberries, or yoghurt (although I limited these to two daily).

I used to drink masses of milk, but now it was a much smaller glass. I had treat days on Saturday nights with a small chocolate bar or small dessert from the supermarket.

I also started making a lot more food from scratch and experimenting with what I was having to make it healthier and to keep me fuller for longer. I was constantly on food websites, watching the food channel on TV and reading magazines about food to get ideas. I tried most things. Some worked out and were tasty, whereas some did not, and I didn't make them again.

Previously, I drank a lot of diluting juice and fizzy drinks, but I became involved with this water stuff. I have a water bottle most places I go and have been challenging myself to drink throughout the day. I admit some days are trickier than others.

My fruit and vegetable intake increased as I tried my hardest to 'eat the rainbow', which meant lots of different varieties of fruit and vegetables, from fresh to frozen, to canned to dried, then from apples to broccoli, and grapes to carrots.

## Portion Sizes and Alcohol

I made a massive change to my portion sizes and ate much smaller servings of the foods I was eating.

With alcohol, I was never a big drinker, but over my weight loss journey, I cut back even further to a point where I stopped altogether. I didn't need those empty calories.

There was one point on my journey when I dropped my calories so much that I caused my body to go into starvation mode, and my weight loss plateaued. It took some time to figure out what I had done, but by writing it down, I could see it all clearly. A couple of changes to calorie intake and a few more protein ideas and I was back on track in the ever-changing journey to my goal.

## Plate Size

You may think this is a bit weird, but stick with me as I explain. From the 1940s to 2019 (when I did this research), portions had become, in my opinion, out of control.

According to the internet, the plate size in 1940 was about nine inches, and by 2009, it was a massive 12 inches. That is a three-inch difference or about the size of your credit card.

That's just crazy! So, the long and the short of it was that my portion sizes had to come down dramatically, and they did just that, simply by changing to a smaller plate.

## Meal times

My most significant change during my journey was when I ate my meals. Before the weight loss journey, I would eat two to three meals a day, whereas I began to eat four, which meant that my metabolism continued to work. The old way of eating was not effective and meant as much as I exercised, my weight didn't really move anywhere.

You need to have a working metabolism to have a successful weight loss journey, or your body will go into starvation mode, where it holds on to food if it doesn't know when the next meal time is. A long time between meals slows the whole process. The timings now consisted of three main meals and a snack or two.

## The BMI Chart

I mentioned the BMI thing earlier and you may have thought at the time there was more to tell. So, let's go back to this while I explain.

As you are probably discovering, it is a bugbear of mine, and BMI and I are most definitely not friends. I firmly believe that the whole ridiculous equation needs to be looked at. To me, it's a load of nonsense (although I am aware it factors heavily in a medical setting). It has been the bane of my life, the cause of my anger and the difficulty in my weight loss journey.

After this IVF journey, I never, let me say that again, NEVER wish to see it again! There, I said it!

BMI, or to give it its Sunday name, Body Mass Index, is a numerical value of your weight in relation to your height. You can use a formula to work out the actual BMI result. It is scary-looking and far more advanced than the basic $2 + 2 = 4$ sum.

Those who hate maths should quickly turn the page to the next part of the story.

The formula is:

$$BMI = weight\ (kg)\ /\ height^2\ (meters)$$

See, I told you it looked scary!

To make up for that scary-looking sum, someone gave BMI one of those colourful graphs to show you which box you may fit into. Now, if you know me, then you will know that I absolutely hate being put into 'a box'. I do not fit into a perfectly moulded shape that someone else has created.

The BMI graph has always annoyed me and seems to crop up everywhere you look. Having sat in the obese category on more than one occasion, I know a thing or two about it. However, this is where it gets interesting. My legs and arms are pretty muscular from exercising with heavy weights in the gym, but my stomach is where I carry most of my fat.

With hindsight, the PCOS and endometriosis were not helping matters. I would be the average apple or pear shape if I had to pick some fruit to tell you how my body looks.

The whole BMI topic is a hotly debated one, and it annoys me greatly as I don't think it considers people who work in sports or fitness when calculating it. I'm sure there are also other

47

industries that can get into hot water with it too, but considering I work in fitness, I'll pick that one.

Let me explain with an example or two. Take a rugby, football, or rowing team, for example. These guys and girls will train up to seven days a week for several hours each day. They will work on their cardio, lift weights down the gym, ensure their core is up to scratch, and work hard to achieve their body strength, enabling them to win the match or the race. Half of them will be in the obese or overweight category on this crazy scale.

Let's further the example. Take an imaginary man, Stuart, who is six feet tall and weighs 16 stone. He is built of solid muscle, and he has very little fat. He is also in the best shape of his life. Stuart's BMI would be 30, making him obese.

Just so it's fair, let's also take an imaginary woman, Shona, who is five foot three tall, weighs in at 12.5 stone, and is also in the best shape of her life. The BMI results would be 30, which again pops her into the obese category.

Do you see where I'm coming from? Stuart and Shona are the fittest they can be, but because muscle weighs more than fat, they are in the obese category, even though they are not obese. I hope this makes sense.

What annoyed me even more was when I went on to check my BMI on the NHS website. I understood the first part of putting in my height and weight, but the second part on exercise levels really got me.

## The NHS Exercise Definition

**Inactive:** Less than 30 minutes a week
**Moderately Active:** 30 to 60 minutes a week
**Active:** 60 to 150 minutes a week

Now I understand the numbers, and note, this is the bare minimum of weekly exercise. This comes down to 30 minutes of exercise five days a week. In my opinion, you should aim for more than 150 minutes a week.

Now, being a personal trainer and doing my own workouts, I'm nowhere near any of those numbers. My exercise in minutes for the week doesn't have a box (see, I told you I don't like boxes).

Depending on my work, I average between 500-800 minutes of exercise a week, so I'm several times over the 'average'.

Now, it has been said that exercise in a 24-hour period is four per cent of your day. Four per cent? Is that it? Let me put this another way. It is an hour a day. A day!

Let me break this down even further (well, I did research after all). A whole week has seven days in it, which breaks down to 168 hours, and finally, taking it one step further to 1,080 minutes.

What I am trying to say is 30 minutes of exercise and four per cent of exercise is very doable.

So, you can see why 30 minutes of exercise is a very achievable figure as the bare minimum.

The 60 minutes are starting to push boundaries, but the 150 minutes are beginning to push things.

After further research into BMI and those ridiculous numbers for exercise, I decided to devise my own numbers that may help people in the journey of weight loss.

## My New Exercise Chart

**Beginners:** 0-150 minutes a week
**Active:** 150-300 minutes a week
**Extremely Active:** 300-500 minutes a week
**Challengers:** 1,000 minutes and beyond a week

Let's give the people who are constantly moving their own category and a pat on the back to say well done. Let's carry on being active. As adults, we forget to say well done to ourselves on any achievement, however big or small. So, let's take a minute here and just say well done to us.

Anyway, back to my point on exercise. I broke the findings down even further to help you.

To get to over 150 minutes to 500 minutes is more challenging, but by doing simple things such as walking 60 minutes on those five days, you're at 300 minutes before you know it.

Add an average gym class at 45 minutes per class, and then the numbers increase.

In my book, it really is that simple.

I will point out here that I come from an active background where I want those high numbers.

There are, of course, people who are wondering how to get from the couch to 500 minutes, and my advice is to take it easy. Start with a ten-minute walk around the block on three different days, then build, build, build.

I can break it down even further (I did a lot of research!) by going into what are called activities of daily living. These are activities you can do on a day-to-day basis without any gym kit or even a gym to work out in.

## Simple Activities:

- Walking to the bus stop or corner shop
- Parking at the other end of the supermarket if you are only buying an item or two
- Taking the stairs at work or in a department store rather than the lift
- Using the stairs on the London Underground if you feel ambitious. Now, those steps are massively long!
- Sitting down and standing up during an advert break on television
- Getting up from your chair to make a cup of tea every hour
- Vacuuming your house from top to bottom
- Getting up from your seat at work and walking over to a colleague's desk rather than emailing, phoning or texting them

## These Can:

Despite being simple everyday things, with their impact, they can help you:

- Lose weight
- Tone muscles
- Stop heart disease
- Lower cholesterol
- Help your mental health
- Help you sleep better

The list could go on and on, but my point is:

## What's not to love about being active?

# Chapter 7
## My Exercise Challenges

I DO LOVE a fitness challenge. Under my belt I already had several charity bike rides, a marathon in my garden (yes, I did that, too), hill walking, box jumping at the gym, and many more. This one takes things to the next level, though.

After I had done the initial research for the BMI, I set out to prove a point, to me mainly, but also in the hope that the NHS BMI and exercise guru may think again before putting down such ridiculous numbers.

I decided that for one month, I would go above and beyond the 150 minutes a week number and do 1,000 minutes of exercise in the week.

This roughly translates as two and a half hours of exercise every day.

It seemed like a lot, but if you break it down even further and, say, walk both to and from work and go for a stroll at lunchtime, you can easily do an hour with just that. It really boosts your mental and physical wellbeing.

Add in an hour's gym class, and you have two hours.

If you spend the last 30 minutes in the garden mowing the lawn, that is two and a half hours done.

Say, on the weekend, you go for a five-hour walk (during the summer of 2022, I was regularly doing this) in one of Scotland's national parks, and then you have a bank of additional hours.

And so on. It's a challenge, after all, and is meant to be hard.

One of my biggest targets through the challenge was 1,042 minutes of exercise in a week. I did this by a variety of things. Indoor cycling, dance, circuits, and body weights in the form of classes, but above that, I was on the treadmill, cross trainer, or walking. I also did some gardening to help me along.

The bottom line to these exercise minutes is, yes, there is a chart, but the main element, which is far superior to the chart is:

Drum roll please:

**Just Get Active!**

Do just that.

You don't necessarily have to get to my challenge of 1,000 minutes a week, but challenge yourself personally and aim for an extra hour or two.

Start from there and see what happens. Believe me when I say your mind, mental health, physical health, and general well-being will all thank you.

Along the way, you may lose weight, tone up those muscles, improve your posture, speak to people at the gym and make friends, hang out with your favourite person, and so on.

# Chapter 8
## Goodbye Weights, But I Still Love You

WHEN I JOINED a new gym, part of the introductory offer included a chat with a nutritionist about my eating habits. She went through what I had been eating, popped me on a funny-looking machine and then we chatted. Said machine sent an electrical signal through my body to measure fat, muscle, calorie expenditure and biological age. It provided a lot of interesting answers, to say the least. My personal favourite was backing up the fact that I think a BMI measurement on me is useless.

However, and this is the issue, it takes your full weight. It takes your fat, blood, water, muscle, bone and all that other stuff in our bodies that make it work. It doesn't separate it.

And this is where I fell down. At this point, I had lost around eight kilos, which was probably fat-based. I still had to lose another ten kilos to reach the IVF criteria BMI number. But, and this was a big but, due to that magic nutritionist machine I could only lose a further four (ish) kilos in fat. So, what about the six other kilos? I hear you cry. Muscle. To get to the IVF number, I was now having to lose healthy muscle.

As a female, I am quite muscular and strong. I love lifting weights. Getting into those big squat racks in the gym and lifting are my personal bests. I love doing deadlift moves from the floor with big Olympic bars, feeling the burn of a bicep curl in the free weight section, and my absolute favourite is feeling the DOMS (delayed onset muscle soreness) post-workout. I was strong, and I loved it. But I would have to stop and be careful of what I was lifting going forwards.

After years of doing heavy weights, I had to give it a break and concentrate on cardio to decrease muscle mass. Dance classes and boxing are thankfully cardio-based exercises, but I would also have to try this running thing again. As I have said, running and I are not the best friends. The first time I attempted running, I got so far and then had my appendix out. The second time I tried it, I slipped a disc in my back. After that, I hung up my running shoes as I wasn't about to attempt a third time.

However, here I was, having to attempt a round three. I hoped with a gradual build into it and a physio on standby, the third time would be better.

Let's just say that running thing lasted about a week for me. I mean, why do something that you hate doing! I have a local running track near my house and went there one Sunday morning to try it out. I'd like to say it was great, but it was awful. It was cold, tipping it down with rain, the ground had so many puddles on it, and it was an early Sunday morning. I was very tempted to take a photograph of this and send it to my IVF consultant with a note saying, 'This is weight loss'.

I started slowly and just let my legs take me where I needed to go. I ran around 4.4 km, which was a triumph in itself, but I hated every minute of it. I had not run like that in about 18 months, so I thought it was a good attempt, but it was not something I wanted to repeat, especially not at silly o'clock on a Sunday morning when my bed and the cartoon channel were calling.

During my weight loss journey, I sought some help from nutritionists. Now, as a personal trainer, I had the basics of nutrition, but it was becoming clear that I needed some expert advice to help with this tricky and frustrating problem.

The first nutritionist at my local gym was a nice woman who helped me by explaining the BMI situation and telling me to eat more protein. It was worth a try as I was still stuck on the same weight and had been for a few months. I did some research and came across a variety of different people.

Off went a few emails. One came back from somebody with a background in autoimmune conditions. I thought it was worth a shot and toddled over to see her.

An hour and a half later, once we had scrutinised my food diary, exercise, and medical history, we had a conclusion and some further ideas. Some of them made perfect sense, and some of them were a bit 'out there'.

According to this nutritionist, endometriosis is like an autoimmune disorder, which means the body gets confused and starts attacking the healthy cells. Endometriosis is also an inflammatory condition, which is why it is likened to an autoimmune disorder.

For me, there is inflammation around the ovaries and the womb, and that is where half of my problems lie. There is still a lot of research to be done on this idea, but I am sure in time there will be more information.

But what did this mean for me? Well, in simple terms, it meant I had a  10-foot fire inside of me when it should have been around the one to 2-foot mark. The foods I ate increased the fire to 20 or 30 feet. This, in turn, inflamed my body, preventing it from recovering. However, and here was the good news. If I changed the food I ate, I could bring down this fire to one foot. Just by eating a different diet, I could make the change so the fire would burn at one foot rather than thirty feet. Now, that was a brain puzzle!

Her recommendations had several different elements to help. The first was to give up dairy-based products, and the second was to give up all gluten-based products. Not only to give up gluten but also to be aware that any contaminates could be enough to raise the inflammation levels.

Let me explain that last point a little better. Normal porridge oats are gluten-free, but they hang out in a field where wheat could have been and get contaminated.

The third advice point was to give up soya. I was already intolerant to it, so this was easy.

The downside was that a lot of gluten-free and dairy-free products had soya-based products in them to counteract them all. I would be doing a lot of cooking from scratch, but that was the way it had to be done. Becoming dairy, gluten, and soya-free would help to reduce the inflammation markers in my body.

She didn't stop there either. The other advice was to make sure that I finished eating by seven o'clock in the evening and had a better bedtime routine involving Epsom salts. The Epsom salts would help take the toxins out of my body which is good, and I would also feel sleepy after doing this.

I had to eat lots more fruit and vegetables to make sure I was getting the right vitamins and nutrients. I also had to eat flaxseed daily and add anti-inflammatory foods like ginger, garlic, and turmeric to smoothies. All of this would help bring down the inflammation surrounding my insides. Drinking more water was on the cards as well. Eating pork and any processed foods was out. So, no more bacon, sausages, and ham sandwiches.

The sugar and protein monsters were also part of the story. Removing more processed foods would mean a lot less sugar going through me. I was still allowed dark chocolate but had to watch my proteins. From what I understood, the sugar monster runs around the body, causing havoc. Once protein has been consumed, it eats the sugar monsters. The body then has to find other sources to snack on, which would be my fat. This would, in turn, make me lose weight.

There was also the inflammation surrounding my ovaries. Oestrogen in my body was being a bully and inflaming my ovaries and womb. But here was the good news. If I could change my diet, it would bring down the inflammation surrounding my ovaries, allowing them to work better. There was some suggestion this might also reduce the need for another emergency surgery to deal with the ovarian cysts. There was then the hope that if there were a good egg in one of my ovaries, it would be looked after by the oestrogen. They would become friends rather than enemies. This might even be the egg that allowed me to have a child.

Bearing in mind that I had been on my weight loss journey for the last several months and had now stalled, I wasn't expecting an easy ride or solution to get everything back on track. I was used to hard work, and the one-step forwards, three-step backwards approach, and the answer to this was no different. I was going to need more hard work and another diet re-vamp. I needed to be a lot more organised when making food, and I would need to keep track of what I ate.

However, the good news was that there could be weight loss and a lot less inflammation, both on the inside and outside of my body, and even better, there could be a golden egg in there with the start of my dream on it. I decided to take on board what the nutritionist had said and once more re-vamp my diet.

# Chapter 9
## Becoming Gluten-free and Dairy-free

FOLLOWING ON FROM what the nutritionist had said, I delved a little deeper into research. I had read and watched a lot about the benefits (and disadvantages) of being gluten-free and dairy-free, so I thought it could help me.

Firstly, a gluten-free diet excludes the protein gluten. This includes barley, rye, oats, grains containing wheat, and spelt. Those people with coeliac disease or who have a gluten sensitivity must have a totally gluten-free diet. However, some people who do not have these conditions find they put on weight on a gluten-free diet because a lot of gluten-free food is high in sugar.

It is very important you have some knowledge on the subject and consult your GP, or a nutritionist/dietician before embarking on a totally gluten-free diet.

Some of the benefits of being gluten-free are that it can improve cholesterol levels, promote a healthy digestive system, and increase energy levels. It may reduce your risk of heart disease, some cancers and diabetes, and it makes you aware of what you are putting in your body as fuel.

I spent several hours over the weeks in the gluten-free aisle of a supermarket during my time to becoming gluten-free. I found that most gluten-free things had incredible amounts of sugar, salt, and fat in them, though not all. My conclusion was that when going gluten-free, you need to make a lot of your own foods from scratch rather than store-bought. This way, you can monitor the sugar, salt, and fat content. You have to change most of what you are eating. For breakfast, I used to eat cereal; now, I eat either porridge made from certified gluten-free oats with a little apple sauce, or eggs with tomatoes. So, from once having the quick and easy option, I now needed to be prepared for what I ate. Later on, I discovered gluten-free cereal, but often, the cardboard box it comes in tastes better than the actual product. However, gluten-free products are improving constantly.

Secondly, having a dairy-free diet. This means that there is no dairy in your diet. No milk, cheese, ice cream, and the list could go on. The main downside of being dairy-free is the lack of calcium. There is obviously a lot of calcium in dairy-based foods. However, there is also calcium in green leafy vegetables, nuts, seeds, dried fruits, and pulses.

Cutting out dairy means the removal of saturated fats, sugar, and salt from your diet, which in turn decreases your calories. It can also heighten your senses. There is a protein called casein in dairy, which can lead to extra mucus production. Dairy-free can also be good for your skin, as I discovered when my skin rashes cleared up and have remained that way.

The downside for me was that many dairy-free foods contain a plant-based ingredient called soya, which I am highly intolerant of. This proves slightly tricky for the cheese, yoghurts, ice cream, dessert and many more food groups. On the plus side, I have found goat's and sheep's milk for cheese, and it turns out I am only intolerant of cow's milk. The vegan cheeses, in my mind, are not the greatest. In terms of milk, I mainly use coconut, oat or cashew milk (other dairy-free milks are available!). Coconut milk tends to help when making cakes and desserts, whereas cashew or oat milk is great for basic cooking and cheese sauces. It means that a 'quick and easy' fix is no longer possible, and I need to be more prepared.

Detoxing from gluten and dairy is no mean feat either. It takes time for your body to adjust to this. It's not an overnight fix. I think, in total, it took me around six weeks to be completely free from gluten and dairy. There were no major side effects either, which was lucky. Over the weeks, I noticed how my skin cleared up, my energy levels came back, my sleep improved, and I felt 'cleaner'.

I have referenced my findings in the appendices page at the end of the book.

Today, I'm still very much gluten-free, dairy-free, and soya intolerant. I have learned that even eating gluten by accident can cause my belly to swell and leave me with a crampy stomach and sickness. It's enough to avoid it at all costs.

I felt there was no need for further testing for my intolerances as, between my various nutritionists and me, we had it under control. The bottom line is that with my diet and the things I avoid, I stay safe and out of hospital.

Nowadays, I make a lot of my meals from scratch. I have learnt to batch cook (make more than one meal at a time). At dinner time, I would make double or triple batches so I would have a quick lunch the next day. As I have said, I can no longer run into the local coffee house for a sandwich. Being gluten-free and dairy-free has a few challenges when out and about, so again, I tend to take my own foods with me. You need to be ultra-careful when presented with a menu and bonus points if the server has any knowledge about the ingredients, too.

During my first year being gluten-free and dairy-free, we had the COVID-19 lockdown, which helped me to do more in the kitchen, experiment with different foods, and see what worked out for me.

I would say becoming gluten-free and dairy-free has helped me enormously, but it's not an overnight fix. It needs to be planned, cupboards must be turned out, things must be labelled correctly, new recipes must be sought, and friends and family must be educated.

I have no intention of going back to being on 'normal' food, but as they say, things can change as well. On this diet (if I can call it that), I have managed to keep myself healthy, and it works for me. I still have endometriosis flare-ups, but so far, as of the time of writing in early 2024, I have had no further cysts causing emergency surgeries.

If you're thinking about such a big diet change, I would advise asking a dietician, nutritionist or even your own GP.

Over the years, I have taken the knowledge gained from the basic nutritional qualification I completed when I went to PT school and enhanced my skills so they have been updated. I have learned loads and will continue to do so in the years to come.

# Chapter 10
## Please Remove My Coil

NOW, LET'S MOVE back to the story and take a break from nutrition for a moment or two.

Why does life have to be so frustrating? I mean, sometimes we are only trying to get from A to B. On the way, there are obstacles, hoops, wrong phone numbers, and people who are of no help at all. You find yourself three steps backwards and feeling down from doing such a simple task.

I could talk about customer service, or the lack of it, for hours and hours. However, I will keep this point short. Having worked in many customer service roles, I have a fair amount of experience. I also have a lot of people experience.

In my current line of work, I deal with people who come from all walks of life, from different careers, who have different illnesses or mental health conditions, and different fitness goals and life goals. Everyone in my book is treated with respect. A seven-letter word that means so much but is quite often forgotten about, don't you think?

My point is that with everyone I meet, I try to display professionalism, friendliness, and a quirky sense of humour. The bottom line is that, in my book, everyone is treated the same. I try to provide the best customer service that I can.

I struggle when I have a big problem and no one in a customer service role is ready to help me. Maybe I'm asking too much, but then again, maybe I'm not.

Now I have set up the back story, let me paint you the picture! There is a test I needed to do for the IVF criteria and it is something called an HyCoSy scan. This is where the doctor injects dye into your fallopian tubes to see how well they are working. To do this, I needed to have the coil removed at my local GP practice.

First, I called my local GP, but they apparently didn't do such things. I was given another number to phone. But that number wasn't recognised. I then got on to the internet and searched for other practices in the area that could help me. But there were no phone numbers that I could see on any website to help. I got one number and gave it a try, but again, no, they stopped doing coil removal earlier that year. I was given yet another number.

My poor phone was beginning to wonder what it had done to be calling so many different people. At last, I got through to the last number, and the woman asked if I had spoken to my GP. In exasperation, I replied,

"I have, and they don't do it. I've been sent on a wild goose chase. Can you help?"

After a few questions and asking about some calendar dates, I finally got an appointment. It took about an hour to do that, but I finally made it to the end. And here is my point. Did it really have to be that challenging to do such a simple thing?

To me, this was just another hoop I needed to get through, with a few obstacles thrown in. It's like I was being tested to make sure I was ready to progress down the children route via IVF. It was frustrating, challenging, and darn right annoying as well. To do something so simple, which was to have children of my own, I needed to go through many, many hoops.

The words 'what else do they want from me' seemed to be a recurring theme during the IVF process. I'd changed my diet, changed it again and finally changed it so it made even more sense. I now ate a lot more than I did. The first few weeks were nerve-racking and scary while I looked at the amount I had to get through. Now, I was willingly making my own breakfasts and lunches to ensure I had the correct meals and snacks. And I could now admit that I do like to snack. My appetite was back, and I was not 'hangry' as often. We discovered that I had more muscle than fat, and that was what made my BMI and weight loss more challenging.

I changed my exercise regime and now dabbled with running. Running! I did many more gym classes. In the rain, the sun, and the cold, I trained. I did exercise when what I really wanted to do was to sit on the couch and eat cake. I did my own research into how best to go forwards with IVF. I rang many different people to try and get an answer. I became a massive internet search fan as well. I read articles, forums and much more just to see if there was anything else I could do apart from wait.

Now, I knew in the end it would all be worthwhile, but I was also aware I was going through many different hoops. A lot of hoops before I even got to the massive ones that IVF would throw at me. I knew I would have a little rant and then pick myself up and carry on. I had a goal to achieve, and I would try my hardest to get there.

Then, it all went a bit pear-shaped.

In December 2019, I had one of those fun weeks when I had tickets to the cinema on a Monday evening to see a live performance streamed from London's West End, had tickets to go and see a Christmas show rescheduled from October, a dinner out with friends and a day of ice climbing was for Friday. I had a weekend away booked, too. On top of that, I had PT booked at the gym, many dance classes, some of my favourite clients where I worked and a routine that would have made the week amazing. It was going to be an awesome week.

But…

What I got was four keyhole marks on the abdomen, two jab marks on my elbow from where I had blood taken, one in my hand from an IV drip, and a further one in my bum from medicine. If you haven't guessed already, I had another emergency surgery on my ovaries.

I had woken up on the Monday in the wee small hours with my ovaries playing tennis (pain), took some painkillers and went back to sleep. I woke a little later in the morning to a non-existent appetite. Not thinking too much at this point, I ate what I could for breakfast and toddled off to work in Glasgow. Later in the afternoon, I felt sick and had a sore stomach. After lunch, I felt even worse than I had previously.

Alarm bells were starting to ring as I had had similar symptoms the last two years when this had happened.

I called my girlfriend and warned her that something wasn't right. Then, I called my mother to talk things over. My girlfriend came home from work a few hours later, took one look at me and had me in the car up to our local A&E. I was prodded and poked there for a couple of hours before it was decided to transfer me to the specialist unit in another hospital a good half hour drive away. It was getting late at this point, but I did what we were told to do. The consultant in the next hospital again looked, and I was admitted for scans the following day. The diagnosis was a possible cyst rupture again. Woohoo!

The next day, I discovered there were no specialists for that specific scan, so we had a new consultant do a transvaginal procedure in a little room off the ward. I walked down to the room in my pj's, big winter boots and black t-shirt. Excellent combination, and I was sure London Fashion Week would be calling me any day now. With the help of my mother, the consultant had a good look around. Now, considering they had done the finger check for the ovaries the previous day, which left me doubled over, you can imagine my response to the probe. My mum helped me to stay calm, keep my breathing under control and issued words of comfort.

The diagnosis was they had found two cysts, one on the right and one on the left, which were both the size of an orange. The right one had grown since it was last scanned in August, and that was the main suspect. I had mentioned to the consultant that we were in the middle of IVF tests, so they suggested I had the coil removed, the HyCoSy scan completed, and a general look around whilst I was asleep.

Answering any questions, the consultant put me on the surgical list for the next day. I was an emergency but could have my pain controlled on the ward. My main concern was if the cyst was a pain in the ass, I was at risk of losing one or both ovaries and the entire reproductive system. Not what you want to hear if you are at the start of an IVF journey.

Back on the ward, I was told to start eating and drinking as I had been fasted until this point because the operation would not take place until the next day. I had a few sips of water but nothing more. A lucky move. Then it really kicked off!

Within about an hour of being back on the ward, I had the consultant, the consultant's colleague, a surgeon, an anaesthetist, two nurses and two surgery porters ready to take me to the theatre (and I don't mean the all-singing, all-dancing kind). There was a gap in the schedule, and they would use it. I was changed from my pj's into a sexy hospital gown complete with very sexy hospital stockings, tucked into bed, and wheeled down to the theatre. I had the two porters cracking jokes, which put me somewhat at ease. I was taken into the surgical waiting room, and it was the coldest I had felt since I had arrived. I was then wheeled into the theatre.

At this point, I wished it were the all-singing and all-dancing variety. There were lights, surgeons with big cloaks and masks on, a black table, and lots of other machines. I had people moving me, prodding me, hooking me up to various bits and pieces and straps put on to my legs. The porter said to jump from my comfy bed to the table. I took one look at it and crumbled. I was scared. A nurse stuck out her hand and said you can hold on to that for as long as you need. I held on good and tight until I was put to sleep. So, to that theatre nurse, thank you so much, and I hope I didn't crush your hand too much.

Surgery is weird. You are put to sleep, and then after what feels like a massive nap, you wake up again. My first questions apparently were:

"Did I still have both ovaries?"

"Yes," was the reply.

"Are you Tony?" (I had been told to ask for Tony when I got into recovery, so I was just checking).

"Yes," he answered.

I wasn't in recovery for long before I was taken back to the ward.

Post-surgery, the surgeon came around to confirm that I had endometriosis cysts, which were drained and burned. I had the coil removed and the HyCoSy scan completed.

At this point, I asked about the PCOS/ endometriosis diagnoses as I was very confused. For years, I had been told it was PCOS, and now it may be something completely different. It was one of my questions for January when I was to see yet another consultant. Apparently, the thing with endometriosis cysts is they can come back.

Now, the fact they were in my ovaries only meant I had a good chance of falling pregnant, but what were they to do in the meantime? They have given me a jab in my bum to shut down my ovaries temporarily. The side effect was that I might experience menopausal-type symptoms. So, at 35 years of age I was to get hot flushes, night sweats and mood swings. Something to look forward to.

The next day, a nurse popped by my bed to say I was going down for my scan at lunchtime to see what the state of play was. I lifted my t-shirt and said.

"Erm, I think they did it already."

It was a little funny moment in the grand scheme of things.

Following this surgery, I had to do the whole stomach rehab thing again. It saved me hours and pennies knowing that I was indeed an injury and illness rehab personal trainer. This was a silver lining.

Obviously, all my high-intensity exercise, boxing, weights, heavy gym work, dance and mountain climbing were all put on hold, and I was again limited to gentle walking on the flat. Fortunately, as I had the surgery in December, there were many distractions to entertain me and my mind because I was busy helping friends and family with their Christmas shopping.

Normally, after endometriosis surgery, you are not given a follow-up. Still, I decided that I needed one as I had suddenly gone from PCOS to endometriosis in 24 hours. I needed to know what the scope was for going forward and whether I would still be able to have children.

It was confirmed that during the surgery, they had found chocolate-coloured cysts, which had been removed. These cysts were a clear sign of endometriosis. I no longer had PCOS but was now a fully paid member of the endometriosis club. Great! Later on, I discovered I did indeed have both conditions. Double joy!

Post meeting with the consultant in January 2020, I was told that I still needed to lose six kilograms and even better news, I was given an injection which was going to put me into a temporary menopause (yay!) for the foreseeable future.

The reasoning around this was to shut everything down, which would give me the best possible chance to have children as there was no inflammation every month causing havoc. The downside of finding out about endometriosis is I was still at risk of a crisis and still at risk of losing my entire reproductive system. Now, I didn't like to think of such things. Thinking like that would bring a lot of negativities. I took a more positive approach and, so far to date, I have been crisis-free. Long may it continue.

Anyway, this injection gave me a variety of hot flushes and night sweats, with the occasional headache, but I would take that any day over surgery. At least at that moment, I had no period (very nice indeed, I have to admit). I had the injection every three months for the next year or so. Along with the nutrition changes I have mentioned before, every step was trying to keep my reproductive system safe for a potential pregnancy.

# Chapter 11
## The Private Consultant

I WENT TO yet another specialist to discuss my IVF journey, but this time, I went to the private sector. I had decided to try all avenues, so it made sense to try this too.

I admit that you get what you pay for. I got a doctor who knew what he was talking about, which is always a good start. I could ask him any questions, even if they did seem silly. He was patient and spent time with me. A big thing for me was that he acknowledged my girlfriend as much as a potential parent as I would be.

I felt when we visited the NHS doctor, they didn't really see us as a 'proper couple and potential parents', which was sad. In a same-sex relationship, there are still two people there, and both should be treated with the utmost care and respect.

However, with all the facts, our doctor also gave us some good and bad news. The good news was that I had a lot of eggs in my ovaries. The bad news was that the quality of them with endometriosis was not good. The figures he had were even less appealing.

Using the IUI procedure, there was an 8% chance of it resulting in a pregnancy. Apparently, even less if it was to be done naturally with a man. Luckily, this option was a definite no-go for me, but it was always good to know all the facts, and it made me laugh! With IVF, there is a 50% chance. If you haven't guessed already, it looked like I was headed straight to the IVF route.

I had wanted to try the IUI procedure as it is a lot less invasive than IVF. With IUI (intrauterine insemination), the washed and concentrated sperm is put straight into the womb around the time of the egg release from the ovary. As I like to say, it sends the swimmers in and hopes for the best.

With IVF (in vitro fertilisation), it is an entirely different procedure and, unfortunately, one that is invasive with many different steps. With IVF, you need to stimulate the ovaries, retrieve the eggs, add the sperm, wait for fertilisation and an embryo to develop before putting everything back into the womb and finally have a blood test to see if it was a positive transaction. Again, in my words, more hurdles, hoops, obstacles, lots of prodding and poking and then hoping for the best.

One interesting point the private doctor mentioned was about endometriosis grading. Grading? I didn't know it had a grade! From what I had been told, the doctor said my grade was at least a two, if not a three out of four. In other words, not good news while trying to get pregnant. It was still worth trying IVF, which was a positive.

On the plus side, when the egg retrieval specialists went to look for eggs, they could determine the good and bad ones. With the good eggs, there would be a chance these could be kept and frozen for the next round. Again, some good news, but I would not know anything further until we reached that point.

I was to keep working on getting my BMI number down so I could go on to the waiting list with the NHS. That was it. Keep working, jumping over hurdles, trying to avoid the obstacles, going through the hoops, which I was sure made sense somewhere, and most of all, keep hoping. In that recent film about being 'frozen' with a 'singing snowman', the song lyrics state, 'This will all make sense when I am older'. You can't argue with a singing snowman, either!

I was disheartened by all the information, changes, talking to people and everything in between, which, in my mind, should have been so simple when trying to have a child. Many emotions flew around, from hope to anger, sadness and frustration, confusion to anxiety, and a little happiness. It was taking a massive toll on my mental health, and I hadn't even started any IVF journey yet.

It's hard not to feel a bit jaded and confused when travelling along an IVF journey.

I had spoken with many people on my journey, but I still hadn't officially started. I had spoken with nurses, doctors, consultants, specialists, nutritionists, and dietitians, and I've likely forgotten a couple of folk along the way. Everyone had different ideas on how I should do things. One nurse said one thing, then the doctor said something else, and the consultant said something else entirely.

It was all a bit crazy and, in my opinion, something that needs to be streamlined so that confusion can be put out of the equation. It's already a stressful and emotional time to go through something like this, but then to have added stress on top of it isn't great.

I also got the feeling sometimes that I was being judged for being in a same-sex relationship or for wanting children in such a relationship. The world is changing, and these things are becoming more the norm, so I am hoping things will change.

I was getting annoyed as I felt we were treated more like a number than a couple trying to get pregnant. Maybe it was because the consultant didn't know how to deal with a same-sex couple. It isn't as if we could go home and 'practice' (although, at this point, it may have been quicker!). And finally, I felt that I had put in a lot of hard work to get to this point. I got the impression that until you reach the desired criteria numbers, nothing else is acceptable. I mean, it wouldn't cost the NHS anything to say, 'Fantastic work, guys, now you need to keep going. Have you tried a, b or c...'.

I find the personal approach goes a long way in these things. I guess what I am trying to say is, if all the medical staff I came across were kind, held respect, gave good information and had a listening and non-judgemental ear, that would have been amazing.

I remember one nurse saying during my IVF journey that I could talk to anyone on the team. I didn't have the heart to tell her that she was the first person who had made me feel welcome and talked sense without judgement.

As my mother always says, "Manners don't cost anything!"

# Chapter 12
## Lockdown 2020

A YEAR LIKE no other! I had recovered from the emergency surgery back in December, was plugging away at the weight loss journey and was doing all I could to get ready for the waiting list.

Then, in March 2020, the whole world went into lockdown due to the coronavirus disease 19, or COVID-19 for short. We spent weeks and months in our little 'safety' bubbles, not being permitted to go anywhere without restrictions. We had to line up at the supermarkets to get food, wash our hands constantly and wear face coverings wherever we went.

This is just a small snapshot of the pandemic, and you may be wondering how it relates to me, though. I heard from the news that all IVF plans had been put on hold or cancelled, and they were unsure when they would get going again.

I turned to baking, well, gluten-free and dairy-free baking, that was. My happy place was the kitchen—a place where I could bake, cook, and experiment. I made loads of different things; some worked out, and some didn't, but it was nice to have the freedom to experiment. Due to all the baking, the weight loss slowed down.

It wasn't until June 2020 that I had a call from my consultant at the local hospital asking me how I was getting on. I knew I was approaching the deadline to be ready for the next step. Here in Scotland, you have a year to get ready if you are not already prepared by the first appointment to get into the service.

The all-important weight question came up, and I said that I was almost there. At that point, I was around the 91kg mark and trying to get to 88kg. The consultant told me to keep going and that there was now a new deadline in place due to the fact the service had had to shut down during the lockdown. I had until the end of September to get ready and was to call when I had hit that weight goal and subsequent BMI number.

I went back to eating right and exercising well. Although I had been baking lots, I hadn't completely fallen off the wagon, so to speak, thankfully.

However, I had slowed down with the weight loss. This is when I started trying other ideas to see if they would help. Our nutritionist, whom I had met and given me that long list of ideas, had jumped ship, so I was very much on my own. I had streamlined a lot of what she had said, so I was making my own rules and skirting around the ideas she had presented. I was loosely staying with what she had said, and a quick tune-up with a nutritionist would have me back on track.

I tried to find another nutritionist, but as soon as I mentioned those words of endometriosis, PCOS or hormones, I was quoted silly figures for silly things. Now, I am not saying they don't work for some people, but being quoted £1,000 for a hormone check and asking me how dare I go gluten-free and dairy-free and did I know the damage I was doing to my body with it didn't help matters. There was one nutritionist who didn't listen at all to my story but charged me £30 for nothing. That was enough for me to say goodbye to that world and carry on alone. I started my own reading and research to get to the bottom of this. You now know how much I like my research.

One of my friends suggested the juice diet. If you don't know what that is, it is where you drink only juice for a day, three days, or five days. Let's just say I thought it was utter rubbish, and I stopped after one and a half days. To me, it was starvation. There was no fun in it at all. The charcoal tablets and drinks were the worst. Waking up to drink this black-coloured, tasteless, powdery solution was not up there in the 'wanting to jump out of bed' stakes. I thankfully saw sense once I reached rock bottom and said no more, this is stupid. I do not recommend the juice diet in any way, shape or form. It is starvation with a bit of water to keep you hydrated. There are better ways to do weight loss. However, I am glad I experienced this because I can now advise my clients not to do the juice diet.

What I did next was cut down the carbohydrates even further than I had been doing.

I wasn't eating heaps of carbs at this point anyway, but I reduced them down to non-existent. Carbs are the first main energy source for the body to feed off for fuel, so cutting carbs down or out completely would be tricky as it could mean fatigue sets in. Although risky, it seemed to be the correct way forwards for me (that and exercise I should point out) and over the next few weeks the three kilograms came off.

Then, it was time to go to the hospital for the final weigh-in. I had to go alone for this one as it was in the middle of the lockdown, and no visitors were allowed. I turned up and got on the scale, and after a deep breath, I looked down and saw the numbers. 87.5 kilograms.

I'd done it.

Finally, I was allowed to go to the next stage of my IVF journey. The next step was for the consultant to send my information to the IVF clinic in Glasgow and I was sent home to await a further letter informing me what was happening. I was told that I should get a notification once my form had reached the clinic, and it should be sometime in the next week or so.

A couple of months went by, but still no letter arrived.

I decided to give it a little longer as lockdown was still happening, and I was aware that NHS services were running with a backlog. I always seemed to air on the side of 'giving it time' rather than being on the phone every hour of every day.

When I couldn't wait any longer, I contacted the local hospital, which had referred me, and the hospital where I would eventually start the IVF itself. The local hospital said they had sent the letter, but the IVF hospital said they had not received it. Some eye rolling from me and then a promise that it would be looked into as soon as possible.

A few days later, I got my answer. I had been referred, but the letter was lost somewhere en route. A new letter would be generated and backdated to when it should have been sent. I was so glad that I had checked, or I would have still been waiting for my turn.

But it was official. I was on the list for a start around summer 2021. They couldn't give us an exact time, but that was fine. At least I had made 'that list'.

My exercise, nutrition and schedules continued. I did manage to find some time for some fun in the shape of Christmas, and my New Year's resolutions included things like, 'I will be starting IVF in 2021.'

Finally, in April 2021, I got a letter.

I went to pick up the post, and there was a big letter containing something plastic inside it with big NHS letters on the front. I opened it immediately and pulled out everything that was in there. It took me a few moments to comprehend what was happening, but there it was at the top of the page:

'You get this letter when you are at the top of the IVF waiting list'.

What better news for that day? I had to read the sentence several times before I understood it all and get my emotions in check enough to put a sentence together. I called my girlfriend and told her the fantastic news, and she was, not surprisingly, incredibly happy. The hospital date was set for a few weeks down the line, which would take us into early June.

That weekend was Easter, so I had my last alcoholic drink and sugary treats before getting ready to take the first steps into pregnancy and motherhood.

It was back on to a crazy exercise schedule. Well, maybe not that crazy. I added a few more walks to the agenda, along with some more cardio, and moved my boxing bag into the garden so I could keep my fitness levels where they needed to be. I also made sure the nutrition was on point. No more Easter eggs for me. When I did the weigh-in, I was 1kg over where I should be. It wasn't the end of the world, and it was something that I could easily sort.

I started the preparation and began to imagine what it would be like after all this time to finally get the go-ahead. I started dreaming that in a few more months, I could possibly be pregnant.

# Chapter 13
## The Day Arrived

THE HOSPITAL DAY arrived. As we were still under COVID-19 restrictions, I had to go by myself. Thankfully, the department at the hospital was right next to another area, with lots of chairs, and anyone accompanying me could sit there.

I did a variety of blood tests (thankfully, the hospital helped out here) and handed back the swabs I had taken that morning to be tested for STIs. After I had been presented with a tonne of paperwork and answered all the questions fired at me, I was exhausted, but in a good way, as this was to be it.

I remember asking the nurse about my hormone suppressant medication as I was due to take that again the following week. I mentioned this, and the nurse said I was OK to take it as it would be reversed during the injection stage of proceedings. This was one of my biggest questions, as I was fully aware that my ovaries and womb were fast asleep under this type of medication, and I was in full menopausal symptoms.

I was told I also needed a further MMR (measles, mumps and rubella) injection as, apparently, I'd only had one.

After the appointment, I went back to the GP to organise my MMR jab and hormone suppressant to be administered over the next couple of weeks.

A further appointment was made for two weeks when I would be expected to have completed the paperwork. The appointment would take place via an online portal with a nurse who would watch me sign all the paperwork.

It took several hours to complete all the paperwork. It was one of those forms where if part A was not correct, you had to fill in part B; if part B was not correct, then part A.1 would need to be completed, and so on. Everything had to be filled in to the best of my ability, and signatures left until I did them with the nurse during the online appointment. I finally managed to fill everything in to the best of my knowledge, and I popped them on the side, awaiting further instruction.

During the next appointment, the nurse watched me sign them before asking an all-important question.

"When was your last period?"

When was my last period? Well, I had been on medication for the last year or so, which put my ovaries and womb asleep. I didn't have periods, was the answer.

The second question was,

"When is your period due?"

My answer was,

"In three months."

Needless to say, I started to see a flaw in this plan. The nurse had to find out what had happened and would call me back that afternoon. She told me that one of the swabs needed to be repeated and to go into the hospital the following week to have it completed.

There was no phone call that afternoon, and I went to hang out at my mum's house for somebody to watch over me and keep me company.

The following week, I had the appointment, and again, I mentioned to the nurse what had happened at the previous appointments. It was left with, 'The matter will be taken to the lunchtime meeting, and you should expect a phone call from one of the nurses'.

I left the department with a very bad feeling.

Just after lunch, the phone call came with the answer to that all important period question. There was no reversal for this medication, and my journey would be delayed until August at the earliest for starting IVF.

I was devastated. I had worked so hard. I had asked the correct questions. I was ready.

All of this hard work for what?

Nothing, nil point, nadda, zilch!

I can't even begin to describe how angry, frustrated and upset I was. It was horrific. The hospital admitted that there had been a mismatch of information, and the nurse should have checked with a consultant before confirming any plans for going forward and that particular medication.

I had worked so hard, and I had waited my turn patiently. I lost the 20kg, did all the tests, filled in all the paperwork, attended the appointments and most importantly,

I was ready to go!

Needless to say, there wasn't much else I could do at this point except wait, and that is what I did. I threw myself into work, exercised, and made sure my nutrition was on point. I started to take more day trips. The travel restrictions had now been lifted in Scotland, and I had always said as soon as that happened, I would be out and about.

During June, July, and the start of August, I went to Glencoe and Fort William, swam in Loch Lomond and the like. I also walked. And I mean a lot of walking. I completed my first Munro (mountains in Scotland over 3,000 ft or 914 metres), Ben Lomond, and took a trip to the Ochil Hills, Devil's Staircase on the West Highland Way, Chatelherault, and many others. Walking gave me a sense that I was doing something. It felt like I was moving forwards.

That is what I did: I waited, walked, and went on day trips. It passed the time, which was the

main thing, and I slowly edged my way forward
to that all-important date in August.

# Chapter 14
## Lack of 'Ingredient'

CORRECT ME IF I'm wrong, but to make a human being, you need an egg from the female and sperm from the male. I don't think this has changed recently, but there are now many different ways to make a baby.

As my children were going to be made via IVF, and I already had the eggs, I was halfway to the dream. My missing 'ingredient' was the sperm.

Again, there was a bit of an issue with the sperm or, in my case, lack of it. At one point, my options looked a bit like this,

- European Sperm Bank - nothing
- London Sperm Bank - nothing
- Glasgow Hospital - nothing
- International Sperm Bank - take your pick, but prepared for it to be sent to the Glasgow clinic

The problem was that the Glasgow hospital I was with had links with the European Sperm Bank and no others. All of the sperm had to come from there.

The added extra discovery from a blood test was that I was CMV* (cytomegalovirus) negative, just to throw a further spanner into the works. To ensure my safety during pregnancy, it was advisable to keep me CMV negative rather than mixing a negative and a positive, which has complications for both mother and children

The downside was that CMV negative is among the rarer end of the scale than the positive one.

Again, I felt stuck. I seemed to move a small step forward only to counteract with ten steps backwards. It was frustrating, but I could do nothing about it except, you guessed it, wait.

As I headed closer to August, I had to call the embryologist to see what stage I was at with the sperm. With no sperm, I would not be going forward with IVF until it was confirmed and waiting for me.

Then came the news that the Glasgow hospital I was with was piloting a new scheme in which they were recruiting sperm donors and keeping them on file at the hospital. They had one already aptly named Donor A, but unfortunately, they were CMV-positive. That was to be a no-go for me. I was advised to phone back in a week or two and see what they had then.

I again waited and two weeks later rang back to be told that they had CMV-negative donors in and that the profiles would be sent to me that afternoon.

I had a pick of Donor X or Donor Y.

Now, when you're sperm shopping on some of the sperm banks, you have a choice of handwriting samples, hair colour, height, eye colour, how the voice sounds, baby photos and a whole host of other things to help you decide on your offspring. With the hospital samples available, I got height, skin colour, eye colour, hair colour, a brief synopsis and a brief description of why they were donating. That was it.

The funny thing was that it worked perfectly for me. I felt that I could have lost days with too much information, so when it came to crunch time, those little details were perfect, and I chose one of the donors with a background that matched my own life as closely as possible.

It was done. I called the embryologist back, and the sperm went 'on ice' for me, ready to be used in August.

I must admit it was a massive pressure off my shoulders, having one piece of the puzzle finally slotted into place. The added bonus was that as it was all done through the NHS, it would all be catered for by them.

I decided to pay this forward by donating any bad, redundant, or funny-looking eggs to research. It was important to me to give back as best I could. I also felt it more personal as it gives the scientists a chance to discover more about polycystic ovary syndrome and endometriosis, and you never know; there could be a missing link in there for better treatment and/or a cure.

However, as I later found out post egg retrieval, my eggs were not deemed healthy enough for donation.

# Chapter 15

## 10 Days, 7 Days and 5 Days

AUGUST CAME AROUND, and this time, I was in an even better position to get started. I had worked hard, said goodbye to the demons of June, got my head back into the game, and, most importantly, was ready.

The first question when I reported back to the department was the old familiar,

"When is your next period due?"

I explained that I didn't have any at that point. The blood test also backed up that my hormone levels were non-existent.

Luckily, I got a nurse who understood perfectly what I had to do. I had to go on to a ten-day course of medication, halfway through, add in a seven-day course and then wait five further days for things to happen. If things didn't happen, it was back for even further medication.

Now for the more scientific side of things. As the ovaries and womb had been asleep for around eighteen months, it was time to wake them up.

The ten-day course of medication was to start the lining of the womb to get thicker, which in turn is what you lose during a regular period.

The five-day course was to begin to lose the lining, which then turned into the actual period. The five-day wait after both those medicines was to wait for the period to arrive.

Plan B was further meds if the period didn't come. I was hoping that would not be the case.

I'm not very good at taking medications. I'm one of those people when they have a cold, take ginger, hot water with a sprinkling of lemon, and honey. I have to be in agony to take a paracetamol. So, to suddenly have two different medications on top of folic acid* was a challenge, to say the least.

However, I took it all in my stride and turned the kitchen calendar into my medication executive suite. I had a whiteboard on the fridge to monitor everything and all my meds lined up. It was a good system because if a tick was missing from my chart, I knew I hadn't had something.

The first few days of the ten-day meds were not bad at all. The problem started around day seven of those when I had to bring in the second medication. I felt awful. I was queasy, my stomach hurt, my ovaries hurt, I was tired, and I felt hot. I had said goodbye to the hot flushes from the hormone suppressant, but I felt terrible.

I was trying to keep my fitness up as well, so I did lots of cardio, boxing, and walking. I probably should have been sitting on a couch somewhere, wrapped in a blanket, but there you go. I was so used to exercising to cope with what was going on, so exercise is what I used to control my health and stress levels.

After several more days, I made it to the end of the medications. It was definitely the cross-over part that was the worst. Then came the wait for my period to arrive.

And it did just that. The medicine had worked, and I had my period. Yes, I did a little dance. I had done something by textbook, and I was over the moon. I didn't have to contact the hospital for more medication to bring on a period. My body had responded to the previous drugs, and I had a period. I cannot describe to you how happy I was.

It was time to phone the hospital to relay the news. But the people on the other end of the phone line I was given to ring when my period arrived had no idea what I was to come in for, and I couldn't remember. A message was left for the nurses to find out, and I went to the supermarket to do the weekly shop.

Now, I don't know if the middle of aisle six at the supermarket is the best place to have a public conversation about periods, what colour it was, how much there was, how I was feeling and so on. Maybe the sanitary pad aisle would have been better, but I was in the cheese aisle. I told the nurse this was the case, and she changed all her questions so I could give yes or no answers, making it ten times easier. I felt like a secret spy relaying a find I had discovered in the cheddar section!

The long and short of the conversation was that the period was a good thing and that I could report to the hospital the next day for bloods and scans.

Now I'm glad I only had a few hours until the next day as my mind went straight to the 'how do they scan you on your period' question. It all seemed a little on the 'icky' side, but as someone said,

"You'd better get used to 'icky'."

A true statement if ever I've heard one.

# Chapter 16
## I Was In!

I ARRIVED AT the hospital for the appointment. I had spent most of the previous evening thinking positively and visualising the words 'let's get started'.

It was a busy morning in the clinic, but I sat and waited for my turn. I saw little navy-blue bags leaving the department with other women. I kept thinking that I wanted a blue bag.

Then my turn came.

I was indeed having a transvaginal* scan while on my period. When it came to it, I got on with it. It's funny how the brain plays tricks on you.

Then those words, 'You can start.'

Once I had checked that I had heard correctly, my tears of joy flowed.

I was in.

Two years of hard work.

Two emergency surgeries for burst cysts.

Two periods of rehab from surgeries.

20kg of weight loss.

Becoming gluten-free and dairy-free.

Having an ever-changing exercise schedule.

But I Was In!

The charge nurse taking charge of the appointment that morning remembered me from the hormone suppressant three months ago. She said it was a big 'uh-oh on their part' and the other nurse should have asked the question of one month or three months. I said that it was all done and dusted now, that I had let it go and that it had been handled at the time in the best way possible.

Now was the time to get me officially off the starting blocks and into the race. The nurse gave me my first injection so that she could show me what to do going forwards (an important step as I would be doing it myself over the weeks to come), and that was it.

All that waiting had come down to this single moment of an injection.

I left the department with one of those prized little navy bags full of drugs needed to get my eggs ready for retrieval. A mini trophy if you will.

I was so happy I think I did a little dance all the way back to the car. I even managed a little celebration over lunch with some pancakes in town before heading up to Loch Lomond for an afternoon of relaxation and crisps.

It was great to be out of the 'warm-up zone' and into the main race to motherhood. I can't even begin to explain how it felt.

That memory is well and truly stored at the top of my memory bank. It was great to be able to finally tell my family that I had started my IVF journey.

Towards the end of the injection phase, you get a booster jab, which does exactly what it says on the tin. It boosts the follicles that are lagging behind, ready for retrieval. The booster is usually given within 36 hours of egg retrieval and this is where timing really is the key.

My booster was to be at quarter past ten in the evening on the day of the phone call, which wasn't too bad as it was just before bedtime. The next day, however, my stomach was twice the size it should have been. It was swollen and sore. My ovaries felt full, and I walked at a snail's pace.

The funny thing was I was halfway up a hill on a walk when I got the phone call. I had decided to do as much exercise as possible at the start of the week, so the Thursday of egg retrieval day was a relaxed day, and the Friday was a chill day if I needed it. The nurse told me that I was allowed to sit with my feet up and relax, at which time my response was that walking was good for my mental well-being.

I was also told not to come in with a full face of make up and nail varnish. You may ask why, but it all had to do with being monitored during theatre and making it easier for the doctor to see you.

Now, if you know me, you will be fully aware that to put me in the same sentence as makeup and nail varnish is not common in any way, shape, or form. However, I did say I'd be disappointed as I'd planned a full day at the local sun bed place and getting my nails done. At least it broke some of the tension in the air. Laughter sometimes is the best distraction technique.

There were a lot of things starting to happen, so it was extremely important that I stayed in my routine as much as possible, and I did everything I could to keep my stress levels and general anxiety down for the next phase.

That following day, I decided to distract myself with a trip to the Scottish Borders. I thought there would be nothing worse than sitting at home and waiting. By taking myself out for the day with my girlfriend, I could distract myself with the scenery, cake, car ride, conversation and the like.

I succeeded in this quest and arrived home tired around ten o'clock that evening. It was a job well done. I'd seen parts of Scotland I had not seen before and had managed two walks. It was not my usual Munro standard, but a walk nonetheless.

All I had to do now was to sleep, wake up the following morning and head for egg retrieval.

It sounds easy when you write it, but it's funny how, as soon as your head hits the pillow, you start thinking about all the questions the world has to offer. For instance, what is the egg retrieval going to be like? Am I going to remember anything? Are the nurses going to be nice? And so on. Luckily, with some deep breathing, I slept for a few hours before waking up in the middle of the night. A repeat of the deep breathing saw another few hours of broken sleep.

# Chapter 17
## Egg Day

I HAD MADE it to egg retrieval day. I was excited and nervous, which I thought was a good combination. My appointment was early in the morning, which was great as there was less waiting around for things to happen. My mum came along for the ride, which was a good decision.

The nervousness on the day was mounting, and all I could say was thank goodness I didn't have long to wait in the waiting room before my name was shouted.

I was called in.

All my forms were triple-checked before going forwards, and all names were checked so the little embryo(s) could be identified.

Around ten minutes later, I was being prepared for theatre. It was at this point that I walked past the room where they kept all the big cans of egg and sperm. It was becoming very real to me what was about to happen.

Usually, when you're waiting for surgery, there can be a lot of hanging around in the hospital, but the egg retrieval procedure was slick, which helped me massively as I wasn't waiting around for ages for things to happen. It's all to do with those timings from the booster shot and not leaving the eggs to 'cook' for too long.

The first observations were for blood pressure, heart rate and temperature. My blood pressure was slightly high but was put down to nerves, so I was free to continue to the next stage.

The next stage was the very sexy outfit of a hospital gown, hat, and shoe covers. This is the time I suspect most women love it. I mean, is there anything more sexy than what I have just described? To top it off, you're in your birthday suit underneath. There are no luxuries of a bra, nothing.

There was another short wait after this, and I was very pleased that I'd brought my book along for the ride. I can't remember the title, but it was probably some rom-com one.

Just before going to the theatre, I was visited by the anaesthetists and doctors who would perform the procedure. All the usual questions were asked, so I won't bore you with the details. My main question was whether I would remember anything or feel sore. 'No' was the short answer, and I was comforted that it was the anaesthetist's job to keep me sleepy. Her exact words were,

"The ceiling will start to dance, then you'll wake up."

Well, if that was the case, I was ready to do this.

Then it was my turn.

It's amazing how calm you can feel until you are faced with the procedure room, lots of people, and a big chair with stirrups. Then, all bets were off.

Firstly, I had to go to a little window that had direct access to the lab to ensure my name and date of birth were correct. There was a little credit card-sized tag that would be put on to the incubator, which would be mine.

Then, it was time to sit in what looked like the biggest and most uncomfortable armchair in the world, with the doctor at the bottom end (no pun intended!).

There were at least six, if not more, people in that room getting things ready. I was strapped into the stirrups, oxygen on, canula in, lots of questions and finally, glasses off. All I could do was look at the ceiling and wait for it to dance. I was expecting the Tango or even the Charleston, but no, it just went a bit fuzzy. The next thing I knew, I was awake in a different room with a nurse saying it was all over.

Now, after sedation, you tend to feel a bit dopey and I was right on cue with that. I was sore, but who wouldn't be after your ovaries have had a needle poked into them? The best bit was the heat pack. There was nothing better than some heat on the outside of the ovaries, which felt lovely.

Once I had woken up a little more and all vital observations looked good, I was asked to eat a sandwich and have a drink. Now, being gluten-free and dairy-free, I had taken my own snacks because I knew they had come from my kitchen and were safe for me to eat. The last thing I needed was a sore and bloaty tummy on top of everything else that day. The nurses were impressed I had done my own catering. I had a fantastic conversation with the recovery nurses, who helped me pass the time and kept me calm.

As soon as I was deemed fully awake, it was time to get dressed and sorted out for home time. I arrived in the department around 9 o'clock, and I was going to leave around noon. It was my shortest hospital stay ever with a procedure in theatre.

I got dressed and completed my discharge paperwork, and had a chat with the nurse about vaginal pessaries full of progesterone, which I had to take twice a day, one in the morning and the other 12 hours later at night, to help build the lining of the womb. Then, the doctor updated me on how things had gone.

She had collected 22 eggs, which was a great haul. However, because of that, I had now to be on the lookout for something called OHSS or ovarian hyperstimulation syndrome*, a rare complication post IVF injections, boosters and egg development on that amount of eggs. The normal range is between 10 and 15.

OHSS is common when the egg count is between 20 and 25, and with 22 collected, it was a word of warning to look out for. I had been hoping not to end up with that as I knew it could quickly make you very unwell. So, with some positive thinking about keeping OHSS away, I was discharged home.

An afternoon of sleep, snacks, full TV privileges and regular pain killers was the order of the afternoon until the effects of the sedation and egg retrieval disappeared, and I went back to normality.

The first sign I had a problem was during the night after egg retrieval day. I woke up in agony, doubled over, and my belly was on fire, which was not a good combination of symptoms. Add to that feeling sick, hot, and sore ribs, and I started asking questions about what was happening. A quick dose of paracetamol and trying to get back to sleep was the order of the night.

The following day, my abdomen was three times its usual size, my belly ached like no tomorrow, my ovaries were sore, and I felt sick.

I thought it was just a combination of having a needle in the ovaries the previous day, so I didn't think much of it at the time. Regular pain medication, water, sleep, and gentle walks seemed to ease the symptoms, and a lazy day ensued.

Over the following days, the symptoms seemed to stick their feet in, and they were there to stay. I was beginning to think that I should call the department at the hospital for some advice but decided to leave it as I was due there the following day. I've never been one to take medications or demand attention; waiting was what I went for. I went for the theory that if something big was going on, the symptoms would get worse, and I could take some advice.

The day of the hospital check arrived, and I woke up that morning feeling horrendous. My stomach hurt and was hard and swollen. I felt queasy, I was having trouble taking a deep breath, and my breathing was going ten to the dozen. The basics of having a quick shower were enough to need a sit down afterwards to catch my breath. Something wasn't right, and it was a good job I was going to the hospital for a mandatory check.

After a scan and a blood test, it was confirmed that I indeed had OHSS. My right ovary (three days post egg retrieval) was sitting at 8 cm, and my left was 6.5 cm. Now, bearing in mind that the usual size was between 2-3 cm, it is no wonder I felt rough.

The doctor said, "It will get worse before it gets better and if you get any worse then get yourself to A&E."

Great! Her other parting words were that I now needed a chaperone to look after me as I was at risk of kidney and liver issues, not being able to breathe, palpitations, and blood clots. Again, this didn't sound like a list of pleasant symptoms, and on top of it all, a trip to A&E sounded even less exciting.

There is no immediate cure for OHSS. The best suggestions were walking, drinking water and high protein foods. My diet was pretty good with protein anyway, which helped, and I was already drinking more water, so I had started the process. With walking, except for the egg retrieval day, I was out and about. When I said out and about, I was more shuffling around, and my hill walking had been traded in for a 10-15 minute walk around the block, but I was still doing my best.

Needless to say, instead of going home that day, I was taken to my mum's house for the afternoon so someone could keep an eye on me. Little did I know then that was how it would go over the next couple of days. I wasn't left alone at all, as it may have been a risk to do so.

Very luckily, my worst part of OHSS was the morning I went to the hospital. By late afternoon and into early evening, I had begun to get my breathing under control, which was a great help. My stomach still looked horrific, and there was still a lot of pain, but we came to the notion that, in time, it would sort itself out. I hoped it would be sooner rather than later. Apparently, my breathing had been difficult because of the amount of fluid on my abdomen pushing against my lungs.

# Chapter 18
## Will They Count?

THE OUTCOME FROM my egg haul was that 22 had been collected. From these 22, I had 11 that looked good, and from those 11, just seven were taken to the next stage of being fertilised with the sperm. These were put into the incubator overnight and checked again on day three.

The journey from egg to sperm to embryo is that everything is collected, washed and checked, then put together in the embryology lab where they meet and see if the match before being left to develop into the beginnings of an embryo in the incubator.

On day three, I discovered that three of these embryos couldn't count as they had split themselves from one cell to three cells. They could still be brought back together in some of

131

the later stages and result in a pregnancy, but at that time, they were having trouble with counting. I had four embryos which could count and had split from one to two to four. This is the usual way of splitting cells to form. All seven were to be kept together, and a further check on day five was to be undertaken to see how they were getting on. Day five was also going to be my transfer day.

Cells tend to split into twos and then come together to start actual life, so in more technical terms, we are created by cells going from two to four to eight to sixteen, coming together in a blastocyst, and then the beginnings of a foetus which grows into a human. Fascinating stuff!

I trusted the lab that they would be doing their best; all we could do was hope. At various points, someone drove me past the hospital to send positive vibes to my little embryos and hope that they would continue to grow and thrive.

I found it absolutely fascinating that there was life beginning in a lab in the middle of Glasgow. It was bizarre knowing that life was beginning there, but the womb was at home ten miles away. That is a weird thought, but as I say, we kept driving past and hoping. That is all you really can do at this time.

Over the next few days, I was constantly checked for OHSS. This involved more blood tests and a daily commute to the hospital. On top of that, I wasn't even sure if I was to go forward with the transfer as OHSS brought a number of risks to both me and a potential embryo, which weren't even worth thinking about.

I had reported in for one of my checks with the doctor, asking why I was there. My response was that I was requested to come in. More blood was taken, and one of the blood factors was out by .1 of something or other. If this particular 'thing' was out, it could halt transfer day. Along with the OHSS, how I felt could also halt transfer day, and I would hit the pause button until everything had been sorted out.

I was told to go home and wait. That magic word again, wait! The department may phone me and confirm but then they may phone me to say we had been halted. The flip side was that there may be no phone call, and things would continue as normal. They may phone me that day or the day of the actual transfer. Talk about a confusing time. With all that going on, the stress levels were on the increase and with the general feeling of not feeling great, I can definitely say that it was not a good time with the IVF journey.

I also developed a nasty phone habit for twenty-four hours. I was constantly checking it, making sure the volume was up and that no other calls were coming through that would interfere with a potential hospital call. It was a bit of a nightmare, and it took away the excitement of transfer day.

Transfer day came, and it wasn't until I was sitting in the waiting room that I started to believe that it was actually going ahead.

The doctor came to talk through the procedure and also had news about my embryos. From the seven that had been fertilised, I now had one. The one in question hadn't quite met the milestone for transfer, but there was still a chance that it could result in a pregnancy. The odds were not great, and it could still go either way, but it was a chance. At the end of the day, there was a possibility with one, and that was what I held on to. It was a chance in the womb lab rather than the lab, so I took it and went to see what would happen.

Now, during the transfer, I again had to go to the little window which had access to the lab before I took a seat in a big armchair with space boot-like stirrups. Bearing in mind for this scan I had to have a full bladder, I was in for an uncomfortable ten minutes. I had one nurse pushing the scan probe onto my stomach and bladder, another nurse at the little kiosk window awaiting the syringe with the actual embryo, and then I had the doctor doing the main job. This was the first time in my whole IVF journey that I had a male doctor. I always thought that I would find it a bit unnerving having a male doctor, but when it came down to it, I just let them get on with the job. At this point, I had already had a variety of people down there, so one more person didn't faze me. What was amazing about the procedure was they turned the scan monitor around a little so I could see the liquid with the embryo going into the womb. Talk about an awe-inspiring moment. It was all over in about ten minutes flat, which was great as I needed to pee badly.

I'm the first to admit to being a bit sceptical when it comes to feeling the presence of someone or something about to happen, but I think I need to change my mind after egg retrieval day.

The first day I drove past the hospital, I felt a strong presence, as if something was happening there. This was the day the egg met the sperm to start its journey, so it all made sense.

The first day I got checked with OHSS, I felt a much stronger presence as I was actually in the hospital and about two doors away from the lab where my embryos were. This was when I went from seven embryos down to four front runners.

This happened the second day I was being checked as well. On the transfer day, I felt that someone was in trouble and that they needed me as soon as possible to help them out. From what I now know, this also makes sense, as I had an embryo lagging behind its milestone but good enough to be transferred to start its womb journey.

At the end of the day, whatever it was, it made me feel better, which was the best feeling I could have.

# Chapter 19
## Waiting

AFTER TRANSFER DAY, it was again an afternoon of couch sitting, snacks and full TV privileges. All I could do now was wait. They estimated I still had a week or so of OHSS recovery but was deemed well enough to be at home without a daily hospital commute. I admit it was great to have a break from hospitals as well.

Over the past seven to ten days, I'd been in the hospital a lot. I had waited at appointments, talked to various people, had different scans and blood tests and talked through a lot of 'what ifs'. It was going to be great to have a proper break from everything.

When I got home, I even tidied away my little pink folder containing all my hospital appointment paperwork, sorted all the drugs I'd been using and brought back a sense of calm and peace to my home. I think that was one of the best things I could do. Yes, I still had OHSS, was very tired and a bit sore but having things back to 'normal' helped enormously.

I'm a big believer in getting back to normal after life changing events as I feel it helps the brain and body recover. That doesn't mean I didn't talk about it, it just meant I didn't dwell on the subject and wallow in it. Everyone is different but that was what worked for me.

I was very slow and steady to start with and had to accomplish most chores with either a sit-down or a nap, but I put all that down to the fact that my body had been through an extraordinary amount of medication, being prodded, poked, talked to, and the like.

As they say, sleep is the best medicine, and if the body needs to rest, then the body needs to rest; there is no other option. Sleep, for me, was going to help me recover from OHSS, the first round of IVF and get my body ready for the next stages, whatever they were to be. As I say, sleep is an extremely important part of the process.

About two weeks after the embryo transfer, you have to do a pregnancy test. It is done early during an IVF procedure, so you are aware of every step of the journey, unlike a normal pregnancy where you have no idea until you miss a period before you decide to take a pregnancy test.

The hospital had told me that the test would be simple. I didn't need all the bells and whistles that come with these tests. As simple as possible would be the best way forward. I still spent what seemed like ages in the pregnancy test aisle of the supermarket, deciding on the 'simple' option, but I got there in the end.

I bought the test, took it home, and laid it in a drawer until it was time to use.

The Friday morning came, and it was time for 'that test'. It was nerve-wracking, to say the least. I had worked so hard to reach that point and was really hoping for some good news.

The first test didn't work as the little marker used on the test vanished. I'm not sure what happened there, but needless to say, there is probably a good reason why the pack has two tests. It did mean I had to redo the test again, and that's exactly what I did.

I waited and waited, but it wasn't good news. The test was negative. There was to be no pregnancy this time.

It was good to find out the result, but it was also heart breaking at the same time. I had worked so hard through the last couple of years. I had lost weight, been pumped full of hormones, had a good egg collection, and even ended up with OHSS. It had been one heck of a ride, but the result did not go in the direction I wanted. It was utterly heart breaking.

It took me the rest of the day to comprehend the result, and I let my body and mind do what they needed to do. Sometimes I cried, sometimes I talked, sometimes I was angry, sometimes hopeful, and sometimes I just drank tea. It was a really hard process to go through, but it was one that I am sure many women go through at many different times and on many other journeys.

I took my paperwork out of our pink folder and read that I should expect a period in the next 48-72 hours, and that was my next step. Mine turned up right on time, although I was silently hoping it would not appear and I was actually pregnant. I suppose most people do that as well.

I was scared of this period as I was planning the ultra-heavy, painful, uncomfortable side of things as I was aware of what my ovaries had been through recently. Very luckily, it was not as bad as I anticipated. It was sore, and I felt bloated, but I got through the week. The good thing about your period turning up after an OHSS diagnosis is the period re-sets the body. This was great for me as, by the end of that period week, I began to feel like my old self again. I was still tired and watched what I did, but at least the pain and bloating had disappeared, and I was thankful for that.

I think with a negative pregnancy result, it can be incredibly difficult not to blame yourself for the result. This was something I was very aware of in the hours and days after the test. I could have very easily gone down the path of, 'It's my fault; my womb wasn't working, my head wasn't in the right space, I didn't lose enough weight, my eggs were not good after all,' and many other sayings like that. Going down that route would have been incredibly easy, but where would it have gotten me? Not very far, and in a vicious circle of what ifs, was the conclusion.

So, I decided I wasn't going to do that. I came up with my own version. The first was that the doctor had taken the time to tell me that the embryo was not strong enough before it was transferred. The second was a little more humorous.

My whole reproductive system had been put into an induced coma via the medication I had been on for the last eighteen months. It had then been woken up with a jolt and told to get pregnant, whether it wanted to or not.

Now, when you look at it that way, I can see exactly why it may not have worked. I mean, I'm pretty sluggish waking up in the morning, let alone from an induced coma by an injection or two.

Both of these ideas helped me get through the horrible time. I didn't blame myself for what had happened. I knew that I had worked hard, had lost the weight and had given IVF my best shot. Yes, the outcome wasn't the desired one, but still, I now knew for next time the whole procedure, what drugs are involved, how many injections, timings, what exercise I could do at what times, what nurses I might see again, the inside of the theatres, the recovery suite, and parking at the hospital. That all seems simple, but it can be a daunting process.

Had I managed to get pregnant under these circumstances, it would have been nothing short of a miracle. I try to believe in miracles; sometimes they work, and sometimes they don't. Just take life, which is formed by a single egg and a single sperm, to make a human being, for example. Yes, my belief was shaken a bit, but at the end of the day, you pick yourself up, dust yourself off, and try again.

Maybe round two would be my miracle.

I was very glad that I had decided to tell only my immediate family what I had been going through. I felt that if I had told lots of people that I would have more people telling me their own version of events and the like.

I was really struggling with people saying 'no worries', 'next time' or 'you'll be fine' or 'next time for sure, you'll get it'. None of these sayings made anything better. I knew people meant well, but when your dreams have just been dashed, and all you can do is wait some more, then that wasn't what I wanted to hear.

The worst thing that somebody said to me was when someone mentioned to me that their son and daughter-in-law had been through IVF and then got pregnant on their own. Now, again, I'm not a doctor or a scientist, but in that kind of relationship, then yes, of course, things can happen 'by accident', and I am more than happy that they have had the chance to 'keep trying'. In a same-sex relationship, we can try all we might, but there is absolutely no way we would end up with a positive pregnancy test and, nine months later, a bundle of joy. I mean, I know it's a lifestyle that I have chosen, but maybe engaging the brain before speaking may help better than blurting out an answer that doesn't work. That is just my opinion on the subject.

During this time, I wasn't speaking to people unless they were the immediate family, and I did lie to people as well. I had a very big discussion with my counsellor about this, which focused on white lies and black lies. We came to the very firm conclusion that a white lie is used to protect yourself and your family from something, whereas a black lie is a tangled mess of emotion and hardship. We agreed that a white lie would be OK under the current circumstances as it would protect me from explaining things and discussing things at length when I just needed people to understand and give me space and time.

As I said, that was the way I wanted to play that card.

# Chapter 20
## Counselling

I HAD COUNSELLING in the past when I lived in London and was with that counsellor for just shy of two years before I said I was done and ready to go on my own journey.

The next counsellor I got was a few years later, and it happened by chance when I was living in Glasgow. This counsellor was a lovely woman who helped me through the preparation for IVF, the procedure itself, the aftermath and all the waiting. She was the one who helped me piece together information to help me get further on the journey. At some points, it was a case of letting things go and re-focus on the future.

These were two very simple steps, but they involved a great deal of talking and listening.

My counsellor was the one who helped me decipher the emotions of the false start in June,

OHSS, the negative pregnancy test and everything in between. She listened, sympathised, and gave ideas, and she was a great comfort to me during some very difficult times. She even went out to buy a book on the whole IVF journey, so the journey made sense to her and she would be in a better position to offer advice as and when it would be required.

As part of an IVF journey, it is suggested that you have a counsellor or some counselling sessions to help you go through the journey and explore any thoughts and feelings that arise. Usually, the IVF clinic would provide this service, but luckily, I already had my counsellor and was permitted to stay with her. Under the IVF clinic procedure, you get just three sessions before being discharged. Mine was private, but it meant I had my counsellor on standby for however long I needed it to be there.

I have now been with that same counsellor for many years and have no scope of going anywhere yet; we still have loads of things to discuss.

She was the one who got me to understand what I was really feeling.

Throughout my life, I have been known as a 'tin man', turned off from emotion and not interested in any other emotion except for feeling positive or negative about something. It was a very big and interesting learning curve for me when my counsellor decided one day to ban the words positive and negative from my vocabulary. I admit it did take a few false starts to stop using the words, but over time, bigger, clearer and more descriptive ones began appearing. Words like despair, hope, devastated, happy, frustrated, angry, impatient, bored, feeling fine, and not giving in. Sometimes, we felt all those words in just an hour-long session, which was more like a roller coaster than anything else, but there you go.

I like that I have developed these words as well as it allows me to express myself better and have more in-depth conversations with friends and family about it. It would be easy to say that I had been through the IVF procedure, and I felt very negative about it all.

Now I can say something like I have been through an IVF procedure, and I felt that, on the whole, my anxiety levels came down as I knew what steps were involved. I felt tired due to the drugs and OHSS symptoms. I felt frustrated, angry, and upset that it didn't have the desired outcome, but I also felt hopeful and ready for round two when it came along.

With the help of my counsellor, I took a very simple feeling and made it complex. As humans, we are complex beings, and we should remain so. Our emotions are important to us and should be discussed, listened to and felt whenever they arise.

I felt that I now had a greater understanding of feelings and emotions, and I could describe pretty well how I felt about any given situation. I was sure I had a lot more to learn, but in the short space of a few months, my progress had been immense, and I wanted to keep learning and, more importantly, feel whatever the emotion was.

Obviously, I would prefer more of the happy, joyful, hopeful feelings, but I understand we need the angry, despair, and bored ones to help us along the way so that we can learn as humans how to become the best versions of ourselves.

On a wee side note, I recommend that if you have a chance to speak to a counsellor, you take it as it is a great opportunity to chat, learn, and focus.

I think it is incredibly important to talk. It's something that I have struggled with big time over the years, but the relief when you actually start talking and saying words to someone who will listen is immense.

Let's imagine that your thoughts are a bottle of champagne. All your emotions of despair, frustration, anger, no one is listening to me, sad, lonely, occasional happy and so on, are poured into the bottle.

Then you mix them up with a heap of questions: Why me? Why can't I get pregnant like a normal person? Why is the story line on TV always about a one-night stand and a pregnancy, then a happy family? Why does it hurt so much? Why me? Why me? Why isn't it happening the way I WANT it to?

Then, you shake the bottle of champagne.

What does it do?

Well, you take the lid off, and that champagne explodes everywhere, and I mean everywhere. Now your emotions are everywhere and in a massive puddle on the floor that no one can understand.

Now, what about talking to someone about these emotions or questions instead of hanging on to them like fizzing bubbles? Why not try talking to a counsellor, a friend, a colleague or a family member (I would throw my own hat into the ring on this one as well)?

All I would say is it needs to be someone who will give you the time of day, listen to what you need to say and then advise as and when it may be needed. It may take talking to several people before you find 'the one' person who will do that, but the relief when that happens is indescribable.

Find someone who really gets YOU, and YOU only, in what you are going through. That bottle of champagne will open with the merest hiss and be poured into a glass, all making sense.

As I say (and I could probably fill the rest of this book with this), 'It's good to talk.'

# Chapter 21
## Limit the Exercise

MY PLAN THROUGHOUT the whole of the IVF procedure was to keep exercising as best I could. I had worked hard in the weeks before the appointment and would regularly disappear outside for a 20-minute jog, boxing, circuit training and a walk to cool off.

My exercise could be anything from 30 minutes to two hours. It was hill walking time on the weekends, and I could disappear for anywhere between one and six hours!

I managed to keep the high level of fitness up quite far into the IVF journey, which was great, but as the egg sacks got bigger, I was beginning to get uncomfortable. A warning from the nurse that jumping around too much could lead to a twisted ovary was enough to bring down the intensity (well, a little bit, anyway!). At this stage in the game, I didn't need any further emergency surgery to sort such things.

After careful consideration, the intensity came down, and I turned more to walking than anything else. I would walk at least two hours a day and further on weekends. I managed to keep this going right up until booster evening before it all went a bit pear-shaped, and my body reacted badly to that particular shot.

Needless to say, I had to take it very easy in the next few days. I managed a walk around the block every day except for egg retrieval day, as after sedation, even I needed a rest.

Due to the OHSS, I would be walking a lot longer than I had anticipated, and there would be no higher-intensity exercise for about three weeks. I was disappointed, but that was what the body needed, and I needed to be sensible.

The downside was that I lost all my cardio training over those few weeks, and due to the abdominal fluid on my belly pressing against my lungs, I was more out of breath doing the simplest of tasks, such as walking upstairs or even the basics of having a shower. I would need to work hard to get back to where I was before the procedures started.

At the magic three-week mark, I was taking steps to get my fitness levels back up and, more importantly, taking steps to get back into boxing and circuit training. I had to take my time and listen to my body, but every day, I took steps in the right direction. I felt more like my old self as I got further back into exercise, and it did wonders for my mental health and mind. I even managed to get my gym membership re-instated so I could go back to gym classes and have use of my local facilities. It was great to be able to do that, although the first hour of dance class was a struggle. By the second week, though, I was back and ready to go. Thank goodness for muscle memory!

My advice for anyone in a similar position is to never under-estimate the power of a simple walk. Fresh air, being outside, good scenery if you can get it, and good company, if available, are all great medicines for mental and physical recovery. My second piece of advice, and probably the most important, is to listen to your body!

Your brain might be able to take you around the park at the crack of dawn for a 5km run, but what about your body?

That is why I am saying listen to it. It is the one who will tell you how it feels in certain situations. I mean, yes, I could have kept jogging, twisting and turning at the boxing bags and jumping around, but at what cost to my body would that have been?!

At the end of the day, my opinion was that it was not going to be worth it, so I took a step back and listened.

I admit it was very frustrating knowing the level of fitness I had gotten to pre-IVF, and I knew what I could do post-first round was not very much at all. But the other choice of emergency surgery, severe pain and an IVF delay, was not a good option.

As I say, I knew which camp I found myself in. Exercise waited, and three weeks later, I got back to it.

**Listen to your body!**

\*\*\*\*\*

# Food

Now that I've mentioned exercise, I should probably explain what I did about food during these times. The short answer was that I took my foot off the food accelerator and let my body dictate when it was hungry and what kind of food it wanted.

During OHSS, my appetite did a disappearing act, so it was a good few days of small meals before I got back to where I had been. During the first week post negative result, I ate cake and biscuits. I mean, cake and biscuits would cheer anyone up. Don't you agree? I spent time in my happy place, the kitchen, making wonderful tray bakes and cakes. I guess stirring my way through my experiences and letting my brain process what had happened.

Now, having made a lifestyle change, I didn't go too far off track. As I say, I ate cake and biscuits and drank the occasional fizzy pop and chocolate milk, but I didn't go too far off schedule. After that amount of weight loss and knowing what I had gone through to get me there, I would be careful. Having made the lifestyle change made it easier, too. Yes, I could have eaten a full tray bake a day, several chocolate bars and takeaways, and drank lots of fizzy pop, but I knew that my body would feel awful, and there was little point in doing so. I could have easily gone back to gluten and dairy with a soft white bun and bacon with a massive glass of chocolate milk, but the devastation on my stomach and other side effects was enough to say no to that.

I was also still recovering from OHSS and had been told lots of water and high-protein foods would help combat some of the OHSS symptoms. As the symptoms were bad enough on their own, I was all for trying more water and high-protein foods to help sort the situation out. That is what I stuck with, and you know what, it worked!

\*\*\*\*\*

## Holistic Well-being

I'm a big fan of holistic well-being, and use it in my own life as well as in my work life, and I have helped many people, both personally and professionally, through some of the things I have learned.

I feel working with the whole body (and mind) is better than working with one tiny part. At the end of the day, our lives are a complex network of elements that feed into them to make them work.

For instance, if we are stressed, we have the main cause stressing us out, but that can affect:

- Exercise - we don't go to the gym or take that walk around the block.
- Nutrition - we don't eat well and possibly drink more alcohol
- Mood - we become irritable, grumpy, upset, flying off the handle, and so on.
- Sleep - we don't do that either

So, to help someone here I look at the stressor, but also all of these areas of life. I would suggest going for a 10-minute walk around the block to ease the person in, then increase this before moving on to tackle the nutrition and eventually, you will see a response to mood and sleep.

That being said, those answers were from a fitness and nutrition point of view, but what about other elements? There might be things like taking a deep breath to calm ourselves down or a series of deep breaths, writing down our miss-fortunes or things that make us angry and then ripping up the paper and throwing it out to say goodbye or even leaving things in the year they were in (this works particularly well at New Year).

I find there is no need to have that one disappointing element hanging around our shoulders for the rest of our days and then getting an airing at every chance we get. It is incredibly hard to do, but if you can 'nail it', it can leave you feeling lighter and ready for the next chapter.

Deep breathing helped me massively throughout all of my IVF journey to keep calm. At some times, it was prior to a hospital session where I was staring at some double doors waiting to go down to theatre. At other times, it was when emotion became too big and needed a re-set.

Taking breathing to the next level in areas of calm, you can focus on what you really want in life. Even further, it can help you visualise the end goal and result; in my case, it was for a child to be born.

Over the years, I have taken this a step further and tried many different modalities, from massage to energy healing to re-balancing, aligning the body better to trigger points in the body, and 'letting stuff go'.

I admit I was sceptical about many of these modalities before I started and I have had mixed results about it as well. What I did find was what might work for me might not work for another person or someone after that.

I particularly liked the re-balancing and re-aligning of the body, which helped me let go of a lot of anxieties, stress and tiredness. As I say, working with the whole body rather than just a part of it worked better. Also, our bodies like to hold on to drama and/or trauma, and if we can let that stuff out and feel better, then what is not to love?

All these techniques have helped me massively. They allowed me to let go of the anger and frustration around the slow weight loss journey when I felt that there was no hope or no answer to the question. They helped me by getting my body in balance before the injections started. They helped me let go of the false start in June. They helped me let go of anything I might have been holding on to post-negative test results.

I had a session the day after egg retrieval to ensure all the bad vibes were gone and the good ones were preparing for the transfer. It was important for me to do this to give the embryo a fighting case of survival into a pregnancy.

The breathing techniques have been invaluable to me as well. Every time I entered the hospital department, I took three deep breaths; every time they threw a new medical word at me, I took three deep breaths; when I was waiting for egg retrieval, and they said, "You're next," I took three deep breaths; before the pregnancy test, I took three deep breaths. I could go on, but I think you get the picture. I used deep breathing a lot throughout the whole process. It helped me keep my mind and body calm so that I didn't have any extreme anxiety.

Now, a little nervousness or anxiety is completely normal in these circumstances, but it is when it gets out of control and we end up in a pickle that it is no good at all. That was why it was important to me to have my little toolbox full of all these valuable techniques that I could draw upon at any given time.

As I have said, and will no doubt say again, women's health is an extremely important part of being a woman. We have a lot of complex medical conditions that can either lie dormant and be non-intrusive or can cause us a variety of issues. I have both polycystic ovary syndrome and endometriosis and have experienced a brief menopause brought on by some medication. I have also experienced abdominal surgeries. One was for a burst ovarian cyst, and the other was for two cysts on my ovaries, each the size of an orange. That has been in the last few years, so I am well aware of women's health and how it can affect women to varying degrees.

The day after the negative pregnancy test, I found myself on a Women's Health course in Glasgow, which would allow me to become qualified in several more practices to help more women. More importantly, I learned techniques that I could take back to my own studio so that

I could help other women through their pain, discomfort, drama or trauma relating to women's health.

It was a great day, and it was a day that could not have been better placed for me after the test news the previous day. I learnt how to give women a safe space to help them heal. For me, it gave my entire reproductive system time to recover and re-group or to simplify things to let go of the bad and let in the good.

I remember having a moment when my ovaries had a conversation with my mind. It sounds a bit weird, but for me, it was completely natural. The ovaries were saying that under the circumstances, they had tried the best they could during the first procedure. They knew it wasn't the result I had been hoping for, but they had definitely tried. They said that they would like to go for round two, but not yet. I took that to be once they had fully recovered from OHSS and not to jump on to the IVF train within days of knowing the information that I knew at that point.

It might sound a bit weird that my ovaries and brain had a whole conversation that I wasn't a part of, but for me, it was natural and a great thing to happen. I knew exactly what my body needed and what the next plan was. Again, I think it goes back to listening to your body and letting it tell you what it needs to do before jumping in and preempting a result which may not serve you well.

After the weekend, I felt a lot better. I was aware that my body and mind had done some good work. It had let go of the bad stuff, had re-focused the mind and was ready to continue this IVF journey. I couldn't ask to be in a better position than I currently was.

# Chapter 22
## More Waiting

AFTER THE TEST results, I had to send these to the hospital for their records and begin proceedings to get me started for round two.

There was to be a formal review of my file at the hospital where the medical team would get together and talk about how the procedure went, what drugs were involved, the quality of the eggs and so on. Once this had been completed, I would get a call to get started.

I was eager to start but also very aware of what my body had been through already. It needed to fully recover before I went in for round two. I felt I had a good lay of the land now and some of my anxieties of what was to happen, when, how and so on, had been answered during round one. Round two would, no doubt, follow suit with an occasional tweak along the way. Plus, I would miss the whole 'bringing on a period' step, which was amazing. My body would be in a better hormonal rhythm as no drugs were to be used between rounds to put me back into the menopause and shut down the reproductive system. As I say, I am a big fan of natural methods.

My only request for round two was that the hospital either skip the booster shot or lower the dose so I would not end up as ill as I had been last round. Now, that was an experience that I did not wish to repeat any time soon.

So, I waited.

*****

# December 2021

After any IVF journey, when it has not resulted in a pregnancy, you get what is called the withdrawal bleed. A bleed where the body lets go of all the lining in your womb and starts to put the hormones back together after the onslaught of injections.

Mine happened as normal in October after my failed pregnancy test, and November's period was a non-event as it failed to turn up.

December, unfortunately, came back with a vengeance. It was heavy, it was crampy, it was sore, and my poor, poor ovaries were definitely telling me what they thought about the situation. It was back to having to carry spare clothing in my backpack wherever I went and dosing myself up with painkillers.

I carried on as best I could with what I had to do on these days, but outwith that, I was on the couch with a hot water bottle. It was not nice at all, but the worst was still to come.

It was at this point that I decided to contact the IVF hospital to see where I was in the pecking order. My last journey had been September and October previously, and I had heard nothing since, despite the hospital saying I would receive a letter with the next steps on what to do.

I left a few messages for the hospital and the nurses, and it was a while before I heard anything.

Finally, in January, I got an appointment to go and see where I was. Now, as I had not had any follow-up or information, I was a bit confused about what was going on. As it turns out, they treat each round as a brand new cycle, which means you go back to the beginning of everything, including weighing in, blood tests, checks, and everything in between.

My appointment in January was an incredibly disappointing day, to say the least.

I had been in the gym like a mad woman, working on my weights. My reason behind this was if I had more muscle, I would be eating more protein, and that would mean OHSS would not turn up during round two. It's funny how the mind works, isn't it?

Needless to say, the appointment in January was embarrassing as I was told I was 2kg overweight and my BMI was .5 in the wrong direction. The worst part was the nurse, who clearly had no idea about weight loss (in my book), told me that I had to 'just go away and lose it then come back as there was nothing they could do at this point'. Again no guidance or help for someone with two big ovarian issues who had worked hard but was currently struggling with the last couple of kilo.

Well, my anger and frustration levels after that appointment went from zero to 60 in about a second, and I remember uttering the words that I was giving in; it was too hard, and I didn't want to do it anymore.

My girlfriend's response was,

"I give you 24 hours and you'll have a plan."

She was right; before the following day had finished, I had an appointment set up with yet another nutritionist and had amended my gym programme back to cardio and less weights.

The next nutritionist was brought on board, and the first consultation meeting was set up. A brief synopsis of why I needed one, IVF, what my goal was and a plan was put forward. This nutritionist seemed to understand hormones, and that was going to be a bonus.

The plan was to eat fewer calories, more protein and drink more water. Exercise could stay the same. I had to start writing down everything that I was doing via an app so she could check it on a weekly basis and see if there were any gaps or amendments needed. If I fell off the wagon at any point, I would be caught and popped back on track. Via the app, I had to write down EVERYTHING I was eating, which began to be a bit of a chore after three cucumber slices, two medium tomatoes, four lettuce leaves, 16 pumpkin seeds, 16 sunflower seeds, two pieces of cooked chicken. You see my point.

It took a couple of weeks to settle into the new routine, but as I was now accountable to someone else who would check this particular app, I got on board pretty quickly. Add into the equation weekly check-ins and thumbs up for good behaviour; things were finally back on track.

## January 2022

Now, as I have said, my withdrawal bleed was fine. Then it went missing, and then it came back with a vengeance. Now the problems really started.

The pain in January was off the scale, my eating went walk about, and my nausea levels were awful. My temperature and blood pressure seemed under control, but, nonetheless, I popped myself down to the local A&E department to see what was happening with my ovaries.

Boy, oh boy, I do wish doctors would listen to their patients and be more aware of ovarian issues. The experience in that particular A&E department was none of that.

The problem is that with endometriosis, there are no markers in the bloodwork or any other indications to clearly confirm it is endometriosis, which makes things more difficult to diagnose. You need to be seen at face value for someone to understand. As endometriosis was still being researched in 2022, at the time of writing, it was incredibly difficult to get someone to a) understand you and b) to do something to help you out.

The junior doctor came to take a look, the next level up came to take a look, and then the senior A&E doctor came to take a look. The verdict; we can't see anything in the bloodwork, so there is nothing wrong. Go home and take some paracetamol.

Bearing in mind my history was PCOS, endometriosis, burst ovarian cysts, a failed IVF journey resulting in OHSS and periods getting worse with pain off the scale, then I would have expected a bit more understanding. Nope, nothing! I was simply given some paracetamol and told to go home and, if it got worse, come back.

That was the answer despite everything I was saying and the fact I was saying that I needed a scan.

Apparently, I wasn't deemed a necessary patient for that. So I took myself home, and it was another mark in the medical box of doctors who should know better (in my opinion).

The pain increased, and I refused to go back to the hospital. I would liken it to a five-year-old having a temper tantrum. I downed tools, said no, and said I was going to stay put. If I happened to pass out from pain, then I would consider going back.

I mean, why go back to a hospital where you are not believed by any of the medical staff or they even have the decency to do the right thing? Luckily, a few days later, the pain went away (until next time).

## February 2022

Now, I was well aware that the endometriosis symptoms I had in February would probably be the same as the ones I had in December and January, so I deliberately tried not to plan things in my diary so I didn't have to cancel everything.

I woke on the Friday morning and got on with the tasks at hand. My period had started, but there was nothing to report at this point. During the day, the pain settled in, not bad enough to need attention but bad enough to have some sofa and TV time.

It was the Saturday morning when I had a massive bleed and had fainted (luckily back into my bed) due to the pain being so bad. Again came the question of needing to go to A&E, but after January's attempt, I was going nowhere, so I called 111 instead. After several hours waiting, the doctor prescribed some more painkillers and said if it got worse, to call back.

Said painkillers were administered to little effect and, needless to say, the next day, I was back on the phone to 111. This time, they arranged a trip to the local walk-in centre, where I was prodded and poked into the ovaries and doubled over in pain. A call to the local hospital gynae department saw me into the car and taken up there (again).

Now, pre COVID, you would go from the GP's surgery or walk in centre straight to the ward, but no, you needed a COVID test before going into the main hospital. It was a Sunday afternoon, and the A&E department was busy, and when I say busy, I mean BUSY. I struggled to find somewhere to sit down, and the nurse ended up doing my COVID test in the middle of the hallway (it was my suggestion as I knew I would be waiting if we didn't do it there and then).

Three hours later (and man, can you see a lot of characters in the department during that time), I was allowed up to the ward with a negative test.

Unfortunately, there was an emergency down in the labour ward, which required a lot of the gynae staff to go and deal with, so I was put into a side room.

All I kept thinking was at least I was in the right place. I got some heavier duty painkillers, which, by the time the doctor came to check on me two and a bit hours later, I was asleep on the chair, propped against the desk in the side room.

It was decided to keep me in for some pain management and a potential scan the next day. Again, at least I was in the right place, and someone might do something.

After no sleep, I was checked on by the consultant, who managed to organise a scan for later that day.

Again, with endometriosis, these things don't show up on scans or in bloods. So, needless to say, there was nothing to see. I was discharged with painkillers. I mean, I was happy to be going home, but I wanted answers.

What I did find out on this trip to the hospital was it was the endometriosis giving my almighty flare-ups. The hormone suppressant that had put me into menopause was the surefire way to keep endometriosis under control (and me out of hospital). Still, as I had come off them, the endometriosis was now starting to play games. My choice was to either get myself back on to the hormone suppressants and back into menopause or get on to the IVF clinic and see if they would take me on the next cycle.

So, at least I had some sort of answer to a question.

In the meantime, I was given better pain meds and got myself online to buy more wheat bags, a TENS machine and anything that I could get my hands on so I could manage my pain levels at home.

Because I had not been eating due to my endometriosis, my weight crashed, and I lost 1.5kg in the space of a week. Not a good thing to do normally, but in my case, it meant I had two weeks until my next period to lose the .5 of a kilo to get my BMI to where it should be.

The IVF clinic appointment was booked for a weight check two weeks after finishing my last period (they weigh you in the middle of your cycle).

It took two nurses to determine my weight and height because the weight and height machine gave them four different readings. Luckily, I had two readings the same that were in the right ballpark, and I was given the green light to go ahead. So, next period, I was to let them know, and that would be the official start of round two, with hopefully a temporary breather from endometriosis.

# Chapter 23
## Round Two

IN THOSE TWO weeks, there wasn't much to do except keep the protein levels high, maintain water levels where they needed to be and wait.

I did have a chat with the doctors as I headed towards the start of my second round of IVF about the drugs they would be using during this round, and it was decided to keep an extra eye on me for OHSS, but I would be on the same protocol as last time with the risk of OHSS being present.

On my end, I cleared my diary as best I could for those weeks and made sure I had everything I needed at home in case it went pear-shaped.

And, other than that, I waited.

Those two weeks flew in, and the next thing I knew, I was phoning the hospital booking service for pre-round two scans.

Now, if you suffer from endometriosis, then you will definitely know how heavy a period can be during these cycles. There was a point immediately after my first scan when I was wrapped in tissue paper as a nappy, as there was so much blood from the internal scan. I, of course, made a joke about it, and I'm pretty sure the nurses had seen it all before, but it was still an embarrassing moment. It was sorted relatively quickly in the bathroom with the help of some wet wipes.

The womb lining was still a bit on the thick side, so I wasn't to be starting IVF that day but to wait on blood results to determine the start day, which would likely be the following day.

I was given the magical navy bag full of everything I needed and the dates of my next appointments in a week's time.

The nurse mentioned that one source of all the pain over the last few months could be down to the fact that on my right-hand side, my ovary was quite low down and potentially knocking off the outside of the womb, which would flare the womb and ovary and then cause pain. She couldn't be certain, but it could be an answer, and, as you all know by now, I like my answers.

The phone call that afternoon was the green light to start injections the next evening, and I was more than happy with that.

Round two progressed with relatively little problem, and after the first week of treatment, I was back in for a check. From the nurse's point of view, I was progressing well, but from now on, I was to prepare to be in every day for checks (a perk from OHSS in round one).

And that was indeed the case. It was time to be a hospital yo-yo again. My ovaries were doing their thing, and so far, I felt fine, which was the main thing. I was dispatched home towards the end of those last few days with the drugs for booster time. They would boost me earlier than last time to again help keep OHSS away.

So again, the magical navy bag was home with me, and the booster shot sat in the fridge next to the cucumbers and yoghurts.

Now, I was due to attend a lecture in Edinburgh the evening of the booster shot, so said drugs came with me in a little cool bag, and attended the lecture as well. Luckily, my mum and I had driven over so I could 'shoot up' in the back of the car in the middle of Edinburgh City Centre! Ah, well, timing is important for these things. It really didn't matter where I was, and the fact that these things needed to go with me just shows how much I was trying to keep things normal for me.

So that was that. The last few drugs, including said booster, were administered, and then it was a wait-and-see game.

I would know within 12 hours if the booster was going to show signs of problems, so the following day, when I woke up and there was nothing, I was extremely happy. I had got through that part.

That day, again, everything was normal, and I prepared for egg retrieval. My mum would be my 'responsible adult' for the day, and we were all ready to go.

So, on that day, I reported for egg retrieval. Again, all checks of name, BP, and times were done, and I was prepared for theatre. The only difference between round one and round two was the sedative. The only thing I can say from these two drugs was I preferred the first lot as the second lot; wow, the come down from them was awful!

However, the doctors got nine eggs this time, not 22, which meant another tick against ending up with OHSS.

Said nine eggs were taken to be washed while I woke up and went home with my mum for the rest of the day. You can't beat being looked after by your mum.

From the original count of nine, the lab had five, which would meet with the sperm and then be put into the incubator. I remember wondering if nine would be enough. I was a bit nervous as I really wanted round two to work. As people kept reminding me, one would be enough. I only needed one good egg, so I was hoping that it was in there somewhere.

# Chapter 24
## The Next Day and Then Uh-oh!

THE NEXT DAY progressed without any issues, and I thought, yes, I was in the clear for OHSS. I cracked on with the day. I lit some candles, and I sent all my energy to the little embryos for a safe growing time and I waited for news about them to prepare for transfer.

Then the next day hit. In the morning, I seemed fine. I saw all my clients, got gym programmes sorted and did some chores. I wasn't hungry at all but didn't think much of it. I just thought it was my body calming down post-IVF round two.

By lunchtime, the pain was surfacing, and I took to the couch with the telly on for distraction purposes.

My mum rang at five o'clock to check on me, and I remember saying I wasn't quite right but didn't need anything further.

Half an hour later, things really went south.

Needless to say, later that evening, I was doubled over in pain with a wheat bag, white as a sheet, raising temperature, and I felt awful. My ovaries were on fire.

As part of any IVF journey, you have access to an on-call gynae consultant at the hospital where you had the treatment done, so I called in. Well, it took me five attempts to get through, but I got there in the end, and I was advised to get myself straight to A&E for a COVID swab before accessing the ward.

Now, A&E in the city centre in the middle of Glasgow was very different to the A&E I was used to in the suburbs. The characters are different, and there are a lot more police about. The good side was they had two metal seats right next to each other as a bench so I could lie in the foetal position, which helped keep some of the pain away.

Again, a couple of hours later, I was given the negative COVID results and allowed up to the wards, where I was met by a nurse to do intake. The good thing was as soon as I got up to the ward, I was given the 'good' drugs, and although they didn't sort the pain out, they did take some of the edge off.

I was kept in overnight so the consultants could check me in the morning.

The following day, an over-the-tummy scan and blood scan revealed the conclusion was OHSS. I was disappointed, to say the least. I had done everything in my power to stop it and thought I had got away with it. Apparently not. I was (and still am) sensitive to hormones and, in particular, to the ones that they inject during IVF. My ovaries were three times the size they should be. I had loads of fluid on my abdomen, and my liver was in big trouble. Not to mention that I was now on the lookout for blood clots as well.

More drugs and close monitoring of water intake and water output, and I ended up in hospital with OHSS for two and a half days. Big oops! Although saying that, I was in the right place. Most importantly, I could feel my little embryos' energy as they were in an incubator one floor down.

I was given a call the next day to say they had two embryos ready for transfer, with one being stronger than the other. As I had gone up an age bracket over the last few months, I was permitted to have two embryos transferred if I wanted to. As I was aiming for twins, I said yes.

Unfortunately, due to OHSS, I was not allowed to transfer on that day, and those embryos would be kept in the incubator, with the stronger ones headed straight for the freezer. Then, I got an update call a couple of days later. It was going to be a risk as the embryos were so fragile, but as the hospital would not let me transfer, there was little I could do. I just had to wait, see and hope for the best. A massive stress on top of an already stressful situation, but hey ho!

The following day, I was able to go home, but before I left, one of the IVF consultants came to talk to me about what had happened and what was going to happen.

Her face when she came in was a picture, and her first words were, "My heart sank when I saw it was you I was coming to see."

At least she was honest; she was as disappointed as I was.

Now, it is a very sobering thought when the consultant stands in front of you and says there will be no transfer this round, well, not today, at least. With OHSS and the level I had it, had I transferred either on the Friday or the Sunday, I would highly likely end up with more complications and, worst-case scenario, in a coma in intensive care. Apparently, when I had arrived from A&E, there was a discussion with the doctors that I wasn't party to on whether I was going to stay in the main ward or go up to the ICU. Their hope was that the main ward could get things under control, but I would be closely monitored, and action would be taken if needed.

Although not my favourite answer, I did understand the reasoning of it all and would need to let my brain unpick all of this as and when it was ready. I had already had my counselling session with my counsellor from my hospital bed, so I had a few people understanding what was happening.

If the second embryo looked good on Sunday, it would also be frozen for transfer at a later date. I had to have faith that the embryologists would know what was best, and I left to go to Mum's hospital, aka her house, for recovery as I still needed to be closely and constantly monitored, and if anything kicked off, it would be straight back to the hospital.

Now, to let you know how bad this OHSS was, I lost 2 kg and 4 cm of fluid from my abdomen over two to three days. Yikes!

The other thing that was discussed at this point was if there were to be a round three of IVF, then all drugs would be changed, and I would be put on a different protocol, which should mean OHSS would not raise its ugly head. It would mean I would progress as normal to egg retrieval, and then from there, the change that would happen was that the embryos would go straight to the deep freeze rather than transfer.

All I could say was let's cross that bridge when I get to it. There was too much information going on at that point to even think about round three, but it was reassuring to know there would be some changes and I should not have to go through OHSS again. Twice is more than enough for one lifetime.

The embryologist called me a couple of days later with an update on the two embryos. I remember asking if it was good news or bad. Her answer was it was a bit of both.

I had one embryo that was strong and apparently had already been sent to the freezer on day three, and the other that was not doing too well but would be kept in the incubator until the following day to see if it survived.

Again, it wasn't the news I was hoping for, but I was so happy that at least one had made it into the deep freeze. It did end up with the name of the cheeky snowman from a particular frozen film, though, but I was looking for a little bit of hope in the grand scheme of things and that made me smile. Plus, if a little embryo grew from one of my eggs, then I knew in my heart that it would be a cheeky wee monkey.

The following morning, there was another call from the embryologist with the final verdict. Said little embryo was a no-go. The other was safely in the freezer for when I was ready for it.

There was a whole bunch of letters and numbers on said embryo, and this is what they use to determine how successful it was likely to be. I can't remember all of the letters and numbers now, but what I do remember is they were sitting in the middle of the scales, so there was a 50/50 chance of which direction it was going to head into.

Again, I was more than happy at least there was something there, and my round two was not quite finished yet. Now, that was something I could hold onto, however long it took to get little embryo on to the transfer track.

I had an OHSS welfare check the following week to see a) how the ovaries were doing and b) if my liver had got itself back under control.

But, the morning before my appointment, I found myself once again in A&E at the same hospital due to my pain levels going through the roof.

They did all the necessary checks, and the verdict was it was due to the withdrawal bleed. Thanks to both an internal and external scan, they could see that the ovaries were under control, but the liver wasn't quite. Cue the need for blood thinning injections for the next ten days.

I swear those blood-thinning injection needles were at least 10 times the size of the IVF ones. They hurt a tonne more than the others as well, and my poor abdomen ended up bruised beyond belief.

Again, the whole episode created another period of being a hospital yo-yo, and that was the way for the next two to three weeks until my liver finally caught up with itself.

Every time I was in the hospital, I could sense my little embryo in the deep freeze, which was nice. On the other hand, I was getting tired of constant hospital appointments.

After week three, I was signed off as healthy and to get through the withdrawal bleed, then the first proper period after that, and then to get in touch for transfer procedure start times.

That sounded fair to me, and again, that all familiar waiting began.

# Chapter 25
## My Back

NOW, YOU WOULD have thought that with everything I had gone through during round two of IVF that I really didn't need anything further to trip me up. Oh no, apparently, my body likes to take matters into its own hands and throw everything at me at once.

I think what happened with all the endometriosis stuff was that it started to inflame everything on the inside and, with the help of IVF, inflamed everything even further. Needless to say, I ended up with a bulging disc between L3 and L4 of my lower back, which pressed against my sciatic nerve on the right-hand side.

The sciatic nerve is the longest in the body as it goes from the lower back through the bum, down the back of the leg, crosses at the knee and finishes through the calf at the bottom of the ankle. They aren't kidding when they say it is the longest nerve after all that.

Pain-wise, you are looking at pain through the lower back, bum, all of the thigh (back, front and side), lower leg and then ankle to foot.

The pain was unreal. Even through all the endometriosis and IVF pain, this was on another level.

And even better, when that flared, my ovaries flared, just in case anything felt left out. The pain was crazy, and by crazy, I mean CRAZY!

It was on the second trip to A&E with the ovaries inflamed due to the withdrawal bleed that I mentioned my back was at its most painful. I was taken straight from the waiting room to majors and given the highest pain killers available to me.

I was X-rayed, and this is where the restriction between L3 and L4 was found. I was sent home with some low-dose painkillers and told to rest up.

Now, with that type of back injury, all I could think was, 'Are you serious?'

I took matters into my own hands and got on to the GP the next day and any physios who had an appointment for the day. By the end of the day, I had better pain killers and a full diagnosis from the physio (who did find it amusing that I was lying on the floor in his waiting room rather than sitting on a chair). The full diagnosis was a bulging disc and sciatica.

I was looking at months of recovery and was sent home with another appointment with the physio once the pain levels were under control.

Now, do you remember the drugs I was prescribed during one of my endometriosis flares by the GP at 111? Yes, well, those were the drugs, along with a combo of others I would be taking for the next few weeks. So they did end up being helpful after all.

The following two weeks saw me lying on my back or my front in the living room on a gym mat with a blanket. I couldn't put any weight through my right leg, so to get around, I crawled everywhere or stayed put and had to rely on people to get me things. I was banned from all exercise and gym work. Most of my clients were re-arranged into different spots and I had the camera off while I did online sessions due to the fact I was lying rather than sitting.

I got through those weeks and it was an incredibly powerful lesson in listening to the body and taking things easy. At least I had time to get my 2022 tax return under control and filed. Oh, the joys of recovery!

With a combination of acupuncture from the physio, body re-alignment, gently mobilisations, resting and walking I got through those weeks. The recovery was a long one, but day by day, I made improvements, which was awesome, and meant I could head for embryo transfer within the next few weeks, which was even more awesome.

As I say, my body doesn't like to do things the normal and conventional way, much to my dismay. But as they say, what doesn't kill you makes you stronger.

# Chapter 26
## Round Three

TECHNICALLY, I WAS still in round two of IVF and awaiting transfer, but it doesn't stop you thinking about round three.

When I started my IVF journey, I was aware it was going to be a roller coaster of emotions and a stressful time. I don't think I realised the toll it would take on the body when trying to do such a simple task.

When the consultant stands before you, saying you could end up in intensive care, your brain will naturally start asking questions about why.

My biggest question was, am I going to allow my body to go through this all again in the quest for a child?

It was a tough question to ask and one that I didn't have a ready answer for at the time of writing in May 2022.

I had a failed IVF attempt, which ended in OHSS as round one. Then, I had OHSS and an embryo put into storage as round two. Not to mention my back getting in on the act and causing issues.

It makes you wonder if this is the right way forward for you as a human being and question how much more one body can take during these IVF rounds.

I'm aware people go through many, many rounds to get their child, but to me, that number of rounds filled me with dread due to the first two I'd had.

The jury was still out on whether I would do round three because, technically, I was still in round two, but these questions sometimes need some thought.

My other big question of the moment was if round two was not successful, would I go back on to hormone suppressants, which would pause any IVF for anywhere from three months to years? On the other hand, I was not getting any younger, which goes against you as you get older with these things (well, unless you go privately, of course, but still, there is an age bracket). The other side of the coin was that if I didn't go back on to hormone suppressants, the endometriosis would continue playing games, so naturally, it left me with round three being an option.

As you can see, it was a very tricky time, and there were some big life questions I had to ask to help keep me safe and sound.

The one thing I did know at this point was that I was going to be a mother someday, but it might not be via IVF using one of my eggs. There are many different options to look into. I kept having to remind myself that what would be would be.

# Chapter 27
## Marriage Crisis

BACK IN 2018, my girlfriend became my wife. However, sadly, during my IVF journey, it became apparent our marriage was not going well (not due to the pressure of IVF, I must stress) and that things were not quite right. I won't go into details here, as that is not what my IVF story is about, but needless to say, we separated and were soon to be divorced.

It's not something I recommend when going through an IVF process, but things happen for a reason, and this was one of those times.

What it meant, though, was that I had to contact the hospital and check what the criteria were, separating out the names, and then the big question of whether I could carry on as a singleton had to be investigated and actioned.

199

Now, as it was my egg that had been fertilised, I was the one who got to answer most of these questions, which, in my book, was a stroke of luck.

I also knew I had to give that embryo a chance, whatever the outcome was going to be. It was a decision that had to be made from a partnership to a singleton, but a decision nonetheless. There was only one way to go, and that was to move forwards. I am not a big dweller on things. Things happen for a reason. As I have said, you deal with the reason and the outcome from said reason, then move on. It is an extremely hard thing to do, but sometimes in life, we get thrown curve balls and then some, and that was just one of those times when the curve ball came with many bells and whistles.

All I knew was that the embryo needed a chance.

So, I phoned the hospital to check on the proceedings and told the nurse about the position I was in. My notes were to go to the lunchtime meeting to see what the next steps would be. As I said, the egg was mine, so that was all good. I remember being halfway through the call with the nurse saying something along the lines of, 'Well, if you can't sort out the position, the embryo will be destroyed.'

Now, this was not the opportunity to be cut off from the phone call, but I was. I was cut off. As it was an outside line, I couldn't call back. I tried all the numbers I had and left as many messages as I deemed possible without going over the top. Around an hour and a half later, I got through to the same nurse I had already spoken to. She started the phone call with something like I knew you would call back. Now my question was, if they knew I was still on the conversation, why did it take ninety full minutes until I got to speak to someone again? All that phone call did was leave me with great anxiety about what would happen to my one and only chance of completing the IVF journey. An embryo which I had helped to create that had made me crazy sick in the meantime and that I was going to have to fight for was suddenly in serious jeopardy.

As you can imagine, there was another wait for a consultant to call me back and discuss the next steps. Around two months later in came said phone call. It was confirmed again that it was my egg, so my decision and that until final confirmation was in order, said little embryo would be safe in the deep freeze at the hospital. It was then also pointed out that I would need to switch from the NHS service, where I had started the procedure, to the private sector as I was now a singleton. I was given two different private clinics and told to ring them, explain the situation, and then see if they could help me.

Over the next couple of weeks, I did just that. Well, I called one of them and had a lengthy chat with the nice receptionist, got all the information that I needed and that all-important cost which would now be a factor into this equation. With the other clinic I called, I left a message for them to get back to me. This particular clinic was the same department I was used to and one of the reasons I wanted to stay put.

Around eight weeks later, after several phone calls, several voice messages, and an email or two, I got a reply from them. Now, you may argue I could have gone with the other place, but that would mean that little embryo would have a trip across Glasgow in its deep freeze tank rather than a trip up the corridor when the time came. In the first clinic, I would have to go through all the tests again rather than in the second one, where there would be no further testing as all my notes were on file in the filing room.

Needless to say, and, although a long wait, I finally managed to get an appointment at the clinic I wanted to be at, with them apologising for the delay on their part due to insufficient office staff. Now, of course, came the new game plan for getting through the embryo transfer.

In the first meeting I was told by the nurse that I could proceed as a singleton and all I would need to do was the paperwork. There was to be an additional paper in there that would relinquish my ex-wife of any parental right to the child created by the embryo. Something fairly easy and understandable, I thought. I could get this done in the week and then get in line for going forward.

A couple of days later, an emergency online video call came into my inbox requesting my presence with both the nurse and head embryologist. The long and short of it was it would not be that simple. Now, again, call me old fashioned, but if you knew a patient was going to be contacted, would you not get all the facts from the original phone call so you had all the answers ready and waiting and said patient was not going to be sent on a wild goose chase? It was also unlikely that this was the first time a couple had gone through a separation or a divorce whilst being under the care of IVF. A rarity perhaps, but not an unlikely situation.

The new plan was that I had to get a form called 'lack of consent', which I then had to send to a sourced solicitor, which I also had to find. Several phone calls later, I managed to speak to an actual solicitor who understood what said form meant, how to fill one in, and how they were to sign it, as I needed the official solicitor signature for the hospital.

Again, more waiting and lots of forms backwards and forwards, with the solicitor's hours ticking along nicely for a lovely invoice at the end of it all. Several days before Christmas

2022, I found myself in the middle of Glasgow at the solicitor's office signing said paperwork. I have to admit, me arriving in my jeans, trainers and big winter coat did make me feel rather out of place in the land of fancy suits, but still, I got the job done.

All the paperwork was sent back to the hospital, and a few days later, I had my answer. I was good to go. Now all I had to do was wait for my period to arrive and call them so the hospital could put together a plan and then let me know the dates of things happening.

Very luckily, my period had been pretty regular over the last few months, so I knew roughly when to expect things, what symptoms I had and what information the hospital needed that I could answer.

My period arrived, and a quick phone call had me on the list for three weeks down the line. Finally, a result and time to start the ball rolling with phone calls and form filling.

All my documentation had to be re-signed with my name and my name only. I had to ensure my smear test was up-to-date, all the COVID jabs and any other injections were up-to-date again, and my all-important BMI was under control.

One of the most frustrating phone calls I had with the nurse was when they forgot I had an appointment with them and then turned up to said online appointment and asked,

"Are you both here?"

"Have you read my notes as it is all in there," was my answer.

The nurse agreed that I would be the only one at the appointment and that, yes, I was going forwards as a single person. Now, why the nurse couldn't have read my notes at the beginning before jumping on the call is beyond me, and all it left me with was anxiety and frustration. I had fought all the time to get to where I was, and it was such a simple but incredibly heart-breaking remark. Going forwards, I had to make sure that it was clearly written on the front of my file to ensure it was unlikely to happen again.

I had fought for that little embryo for the best part of a year, and when it came down to the final answer, it happened very, very fast. Those three weeks flew by, and suddenly, I was staring at those white doors into the IVF clinic awaiting further instructions.

One of the decisions I had to make about the transfer was whether I would have a natural or a medicated frozen embryo transfer. The natural is where you take your own temperature, monitor your symptoms and then go to the hospital on the required date and time. The downside of all of this method is that the transfer date can easily be missed. I decided to go for the medicated version for several reasons. First, with my track record, I thought access to the nurses and someone keeping an eye on me would put me at ease. The second reason was that there was a high chance I would make the transfer deadline as the drugs would be in control of everything. This was the pricier option, but it was the one that would serve me better in the long run.

The way I saw it, electing for the frozen embryo transfer had three main areas of concern.

The first was what if I got sick again like I did with OHSS. But I had been assured that, as they would not mess with my ovaries this time and just my uterus, this was not going to happen. I may have side effects such as headaches, nausea, sore stomach from injection sites, and hot flushes, but it should not be any more severe than that. That was very reassuring, I had to admit. I had worked so hard to get my fitness back to where it was post OHSS and my back injury in 2022 that I was concerned I would end up with more time off.

My second concern was about the thawing of the little embryo. At any stage of the thawing-out process, if it wasn't strong enough, that would be game over for me. I only had the one embryo, so there was only one shot at embryo transfer.

My third concern was the all-consuming, 'What if it didn't work, and how would I recover from that?' I had visions of me sitting with the pregnancy test and thinking my IVF journey was over.

You can't go through all that I have said to date and not worry about these things. What I did know was that even after everything I had experienced, I had to see it through, whatever the outcome. It was a journey that needed to be completed, and I would do just that.

The number of comments I had had to date about the fight I had put in for said embryo all summed up to the fact that I was already thinking like a parent. That was very apparent in the fight and how fiercely protective I was over said little embryo. I had even taken it upon myself every time I drove past the hospital on the way to somewhere to say hello to my little embryo and that I was sorting things and would be back soon. I hoped all of this would be a plus sign on the road to pregnancy and then eventually hold a tiny bundle of joy in my arms.

# Chapter 28
## Here We Go!

BEFORE I KNEW it, I was once again staring at those white doors and then waiting in the seating area for my turn.

The rules had changed since I had last been in, courtesy of COVID restrictions easing, so you could now come in with your significant other. It was a nice touch, but one that brought it home to me that this would indeed now be a solo journey.

A nurse came through to get me, and it was time to weigh in. I jumped on the scales, and it was the first time in my whole IVF journey that I was accepted for who I was. The hard work I had put in in the gym was accepted, the fact I was muscular was all good, and the slight weight I carried around my belly was also acceptable. I was good to go.

After all the paperwork had been checked, I was given an injection. This would shut down everything to allow the next lot of drugs to start doing their thing. I had to be on the lookout for menopausal symptoms, such as hot flushes and night sweats, headaches, and the like. I told the nurse that as long as it wasn't OHSS, I was good to go.

And that was it. I was officially off the starting blocks and into the race.

The first few days were all good. I continued my gym activities, work, and just got on with everything. I didn't feel any different and was glad I was, so far, symptom-free. Then, once again, right on cue of day five of the drugs, the problems started. It began with a little bit of tiredness and weakness, which was again expected. Things started to go downhill from there, and I ended up with every side effect under the sun and then some. You can't blame my poor body for getting confused about the situation, as the drugs were trying to shut down the system and then bleed all at the same time. Even I couldn't fathom that kind of logic.

Symptom-wise, I had hot flushes and a high temperature, and best of all, I couldn't control or regulate any of it. I would get crazy hot, and then I would get dizzy, which was not a great thing to have going on.

The drops in blood sugar were interesting, too. Even though I was eating a well-balanced diet, my blood sugar would drop suddenly, and I would get dizzy, cold sweats, and a thirst which could not be quenched.

The all-around headache, which eventually settled right across the forehead, was a horrific experience, and no amount of paracetamol would say goodbye to that.

The insomnia was awful, and I was awake most of the night, then fatigued the next day, which meant I had to have little naps and hope for a re-set at the next bedtime. After the first two and a half weeks, I finally got a reasonable eight hours of sleep, only for the following evening to be back to insomnia. I guess we were playing the sleep roulette of whether I would sleep or not tonight. Now, I'm a big lover of games, but when it came to sleep, I was less than impressed. If that wasn't enough, my brain was slower processing things. I was forgetting words and having some trouble with the basics, such as will I have the maple syrup, bacon and strawberry combo or the coconut ice cream with fresh fruit combo on my pancakes. You would think it was an easy decision to make until it came down to doing it while totally fatigued.

The weakness was shocking as I felt I couldn't do anything at all, and anything I did try made me too tired to then do anything else. All my gym sessions stopped for those ten days, and walking, which was slow at best, was now the only activity.

The pain level over three days was crazy and left me doubled over, with no amount of pain killers helping or reducing the levels. There is nothing like being in masses of pain when you're stuck on your own, having to deal with the situation alone. There was no one at that five o'clock in the morning stint to wake up to help me out and, most importantly, to give me a massive hug. The only remedy was to dose myself up on pain killers, then listen to music with a heavy beat on through the earphones in the hope it would drown the pain out and I would get some precious sleep. A trip to my parents' house the next day was my priority for some much-needed sympathy and a home-cooked meal.

The bleed was incredibly heavy and disgusting, and I had to go to meetings and activities with my bag of tricks (change of clothes, sweets in case my blood sugar crashed, water, pads and the like).

The emotional side took on a mind of its own, and I would go from crying to irritable, to angry, to not knowing how to feel, all in the space of a few moments. A simple text message from a friend, 'How are you?' could result in feeling incredibly overwhelmed and not knowing how to reply. The tears were interesting, too, and as I am not a big crier, I found this to be a strange time.

And if those symptoms were not enough, I ended up with what I call black cloudiness on an extreme level. I couldn't fathom any of it as this cloud came in and hung over my head for several days, each day getting worse as I worked my way through it. Now, I had been used to mini black cloudiness from my periods before, but that would last a day or two at best before disappearing, and I would be back to my usual happy-go-lucky self, but this new cloud was on a whole other level. I don't really know how to describe it except to say it was plain awful.

The only thing I could think about was what side effects the next lot of drugs would cause and could they please be nicer than the last lot.

By the time I returned to the nurse for the next check-in, I was not a happy bunny. I got my mum to go to the appointment with me for moral support as I felt very out of sorts. The nurse did the usual check-in, and I mentioned the awful black cloudiness as my main concern. The reply was something along the lines of that it was not surprising how I was feeling, and I was exactly where I needed to be with the current medical plan.

At the end of the day, the previous drugs had switched off all my hormones, so the next lot could take over.

A quick transvaginal scan told the nurse that I was at least progressing and heading in the right direction. My womb lining was clear and thin, so I was good to go to the next step. Even better news was that both my ovaries were cyst-free because they had been left without any hormone suppressants for the last ten months, and I had been having regular periods. With endometriosis, it is always risky to have a period as it tends to inflame the entire system so the fact I had not been scanned or under the care of any drugs for a wee while was a concern, but one that was sorted very quickly and all minds put at ease.

The next step was to be given HRT (Hormone Replacement Therapy) in tablet format and then that wonderful injection again in a few days to keep my own hormones away and the drug-induced ones doing what they should be doing.

I admit that I was cautious and very nervous about that injection as all it meant to me now was black cloudiness. So off I popped with my tablets to carry on with the evening.

Now, here's a question. Why don't adults get bravery stickers at the hospital or even a lollipop? After everything I have just said, I should also point out that it was my birthday that day. There was no sticker or lollipop, so I rest my case.

I was fully aware that my poor body had taken an almighty hit through IVF one and two and then both the OHSS events, but I was not aware of my mind being involved. This time, both my body and mind seemed to be taking one almighty hit with the side effects of these drugs. I would persevere, but I would be lying if I said I didn't have a wobble or two. I remember sitting after the 5 o'clock pain, thinking that I was done and that my body couldn't take this anymore. But then I also realised at the same time that I was almost about to give up on that little embryo.

My counsellor at the time was incredibly supportive and said it was just a wobble. She could tell how hard this was all on me, but she also knew I wouldn't give up. I would feel wrecked, but I wouldn't quit. A few extra words of encouragement during the session and a few connections of dots (one of our favourite counsellor and client games), and I carried on.

I was to take a dose that evening of the drugs and then again the following morning before settling into a morning routine with folic acid and paracetamol. At least they could all be taken together, and I developed a morning concoction of drugs, water and cereal. A great way to start the day. The side effects from the previous injection were less intense, and then I started with all the new ones from these drugs.

I had a sore head, again across the front, which would not go away but did lessen after a few weeks. Insomnia, fatigue, weakness, and heaviness settled into my body and associated brain fog, forgetfulness and trouble concentrating. All my gym weights suddenly felt ten times the normal amount. I remember lifting a ten kilo weight, and it felt like 100 kilo. I don't remember ever feeling that way before.

The black cloudiness took a slight back seat, and I was left with a general numbness when it came to emotion. I just didn't feel like I wanted to do anything. Everything was hard work and a struggle, even the simplest of tasks.

My new symptoms were in the form of sore stomach, nausea and sickness, which I think were related to the start of the new medication. My appetite did a small disappearing act somewhere along the line as well. Now, I am the first to admit that I am always hungry, even more so after activities or gym, and you know something is going on when I lose it. I had gone back to the gym as well at this point, but I was nowhere near my full capacity. Now, it was all about the low impact, mobility, and lifting lighter weights, but the gym is a vital part of my life and a perfect outlet for everything that was going on. It was at this point I went back to stationary cycling as well. It had a lower impact, and I could sit happily on the bike for an hour or so and feel like I was doing something worthwhile to keep my baseline fitness ticking over while my body battled the side effects I was experiencing.

My complexion was also doing a fine line in whiter than white (although I had moved away from the pain-related see-through whiteness). People I met had started to ask me if I was OK. I had already thought of an explanation and it is one that I stuck with. Friends and family knew the fuller details, but to everyone else, it was a case of having my endometriosis medication changed, and I just had to get on with it. The good news is it did seem to answer many people's questions. I just didn't want everyone knowing as I was aware of the trickier parts of the procedure, and in my opinion, there is nothing worse than when you have a lot going on, and it may not turn out the way you want it to turn out, for them to ask how are you doing. I know people mean well and just ask the question, but still, it can also cause a lot of anxiety or feeling overwhelmed with such a simple question. I think the best thing you can do is send a smiley face, a funny cartoon or a cute puppy video, nothing more and nothing less. A simple text to say you are still around, you still care about the person but respect their boundaries at the same time. Even better, when the other person can get away with a little thumbs up, as in, 'You know what I am going through, but I am still around and getting on with it.'

Somebody who knew what was going on in my life said that they didn't know what to say or what the correct outcome of the conversation was. You know what? I respected that wholeheartedly, as they were honest about it. One thing that really bugged me during these weeks was people who thought the stark truth and tough love approach was the best way forward. For me, it was most definitely not the best way and resulted in more emotion than I thought was needed.

I remember having a conversation with my counsellor, and she asked what I really wanted. I admitted that although I was separated (and soon to be divorced), I still wanted a second-in-command to help me out. The second best option was, as I said, for thumbs up, smiley faces and funny videos. The third option was for people to take over for a few hours and for me to be able to just tag along, no questions asked. And the fourth thing was for a massive hug, a shoulder to cry on and a hot chocolate.

Sometimes, the simpler things in life are the most effective. For me, it was a case of people just being there rather than making a big deal out of everything. And sometimes in life, actions speak more words than actual words.

# Chapter 29
## The Hours Ticked By

THE HOURS DID indeed tick by, and the new drugs took effect along with those familiar side effects. I had managed to stop the nausea, stomach and headaches but now had a great body fatigue and weakness, and the smallest of tasks could leave me wiped out. I would see what I wanted and needed to do, and then I would try to attempt it. Even a forty-five-minute leg, bums and tums class left me tired and in need of a rest.

Everywhere I went, I took a sugary drink in case my blood sugar dropped, and I needed to rectify the issue quickly. Luckily, I could control the drop with a sugary drink.

The rashes and itchiness were next in line for me to suffer with, along with muscle twitches at rest.

On top of that, my lymph nodes in my groin were swollen and sore as my body tried to battle what was happening with it. The lymph nodes are the main guys who help your body fight infection or illness. Now, I wasn't fighting those, but I was fighting a tonne of drugs in order to get to the end goal of a successful embryo transfer.

I ended up at one point on the drugs to line the womb lining and then another batch of drugs to help sort the side effects of the first drugs I had been given. It was a crazy time at best, and I was still very aware I had more to come and wasn't at the main event yet. It is amazing what the body can put up with, and if I had been a case study for a medical student at the time, I am sure they would have had loads to write about in their case study book.

I tried to keep things in a routine as best I could, knowing it would help me in the long run. I was still working at the time, dealing with clients, networking for my business, training at the gym and everything in between. To me, being in a routine helped me massively as it was a distraction as well as getting things done. I think when you are alone, too much of your own company is sometimes not the best option for you.

I was checked along the way at the hospital by the IVF team to see if the womb lining was doing what it was supposed to be doing. This meant lots of transvaginal scans along with being prodded. The womb lining had to be a particular 'juiciness', for want of a better word, and until it got to that stage, then the drugs kept coming.

Finally, I attended one appointment where I got the magical green light to go to the next stage. This was one of the most important stages of the last few weeks and everything that I had been working towards with the drugs, appointments and scans, and it was one of the biggest stages of the whole process.

This stage was to wake up the little embryo that had been in the freezer at the hospital at a tropical minus 196.1 degrees Celsius. It would be a quick procedure to wake up and take mere hours. The transfer day plan was to get a call from the embryologist first thing in the morning confirming that I was ready to go and that they still wanted to wake up the embryo. The next

225

stage was for the embryologists to go to the freezer and then start the thawing procedure. If the thawing procedure went well, then we could go to transfer, and if it didn't go well, then it was game over.

I was up early on that Friday and waited for the phone call around eight o'clock in the morning to confirm the go-ahead. It was then an anxious wait for the second phone call to say we could go for transfer. During that time, there was a lot of pacing, and it was safe to say that I couldn't settle to do anything. Even my washing up and laundry didn't have its usual appeal.

My second in command, in the shape of my mother, arrived sometime during the wait, so we both waited patiently for 'that' call.

And then it came!

After years of waiting, tests, scans, drugs and heartache, we were told the embryo had been thawed and was doing everything it was supposed to at that point. We had two hours to get to the hospital for transfer.

Fortunately, I only live about a 20-minute drive to the hospital, and we were there within the hour. My mum and I arrived at the hospital knowing that we would be leaving with a very special embryo safely back where it should have been months ago.

We waited as patiently as we could in the waiting room for my name to be called. It wasn't a long wait, and we were ushered into the changing room where we had to get our 'glad rags' (aka our hospital gowns and protective wear for being in such a sensitive environment).

The embryologist came in and told us that the embryo had been marked as a 3BB in the marking scheme. Now for a wee bit of science before I get back to the story:

The number refers to the embryo and expansion of the blastocyst cavity and its hatching into the zona pellucida. The numbers are between one and six. The first letter is from A to C, and refers to the quality of the cell mass, which becomes the main body of the embryo after transfer. The second letter again is from A to C and refers to the grade of quality for the trophectoderm, which then forms to be the placenta and embryonic tissues post-transfer. See, I told you I liked my science.

3BB was right in the middle of everything and was deemed 'average' in the grand scheme of things. It had a 50% chance of surviving to a pregnancy and a 42% chance of surviving to a live birth. Add into that the additional complication with my PCOS and endometriosis (and general hormone sensitivity), and the odds of a baby were looking very slim. Still, I had to give my egg a chance. I had come so far with things that I just had to give it all a chance, whatever the outcome.

From the changing room, we were taken into the transfer room and set up for the procedure.

My mum got to sit beside the couch, and I had to be derobed slightly and my feet put into stirrups. Now, there was a change in the scan here. All my other scans had been transvaginal scans, which meant an empty bladder before we went ahead, but this was an over-the-tummy ultrasound with a full bladder so everyone could see the landmarks to be able to work and put the embryo where it was supposed to go. There is nothing worse than having a full bladder and having someone push down on it when someone else has a speculum in your vagina. The glamour of it all!

I had already said that I wanted the smallest speculum, but when the medical team tried to start the procedure, I was so tense it was beginning to be a struggle. Suddenly, there was a hand over my shoulder and calming words, 'You know this. It's your breathing.'

Mothers know best, is all I can say.

A deep breath later, we could proceed. A few moments after that the checks were done, and the transfer was complete. It was to be a waiting game now.

There was nothing else for my mum and me to do except keep going with our routines and wait the two weeks till I could take a pregnancy test to see what the outcome would be for the little embryo.

# Chapter 30
## This Time Felt Different

I DIDN'T FEEL much different to start with. I just felt normal for that first week of the transfer, but by the second week, things began to change.

I was at the gym one day and lay on my stomach to do an ab exercise. Something felt different. My stomach felt sore, and my breasts were incredibly uncomfortable. I was also starting to pee a lot.

Looking online at possible reasons for this only led to one thing.

But again, I waited for the test results before I could believe anything. I had made it past the first week and was well into the second week, and the embryo still seemed safely in my womb, but I wasn't going to believe anything until I had more evidence.

Two weeks later, I could take the test.

I woke up early that morning and needed to pee but was aware that this was a very important pee, so I left it as long as humanly possible before going to sort the situation.

I took the test!

The result appeared within the first minute.

It was positive!

The embryo was still there and there was a positive pregnancy test to prove it. But at five o'clock in the morning, it was slightly difficult to know who to call at that hour, but very thankfully, I have a sister who lives in New Zealand where it was six o'clock in the evening, and she would most probably be awake.

So, I rang in tears, saying down the phone that there were 'two lines'. At first, it took my sister a second or two to figure out what I was referring to, but we got there in the end. She was thrilled and couldn't wait to hear about the next steps.

Next on the list was to tell my parents. I waited an hour or two before I ventured over to their house with my positive test sitting in its packet in the cup holder of the car.

They were both thrilled and interested in the next steps.

We knew I had to stay with the IVF unit until the viability scan at eight weeks, and at that point, I would be transferred into maternity services if all was good.

Again, we waited.

I was busy working one evening a couple of weeks after the test when I went to the bathroom and saw blood. I knew this couldn't be good.

I didn't do anything at that point and waited to see what would happen, but two more bathroom trips later, there was a lot more blood there. I knew I had to do something to sort it out, but as it was very late at night, I couldn't contact the IVF clinic till the morning.

A trip to the safety of my parent's house for the night was in order until we could get to the bottom of what was happening.

I admit that at this point, I felt that was the end of my pregnancy. The euphoria of the positive test was replaced with the devastating blow that something was wrong, which could potentially be really bad and game over.

A call to the IVF clinic the next day saw me taking my morning medication before a trip to the hospital for a chat, blood tests, and a potential scan. It was an anxious time, to say the least, and there was lots more waiting.

A nurse took my blood to see where my HCG levels were. The point was that if they were high, I was still pregnant, and if they were low or non-existent, I was not. It was a simple blood test with a lot riding on it.

With my bloods taken and on their way to the lab for testing, my mother and I were sent home to wait for further information. Later that afternoon, we had a call to say that my levels were indeed where they should be for this stage of pregnancy, but the hospital wanted to do a scan to triple-check everything and see if they could find a source of the bleeding. An anxious overnight wait to see the outcome.

The following day it was a trip back to the hospital for a further scan.

A very helpful and understanding doctor explained that a bleed could be anything from the embryo developing in the fallopian tube and ectopic pregnancy, which would need immediate action, to no known reason for the bleed. The scale was vast from OK to not OK.

Checking everything in a transvaginal scan revealed no ectopic pregnancy, and the embryo was still safely in the womb with signs of it developing. Everything was as it should be, and there was nothing else in the womb or ovaries that was a cause for concern. The embryo was to keep growing, and it was deemed no known cause for this bleeding other than, 'It sometimes just happens'.

I was to be monitored by the IVF department and to let them know if the bleeding continued. If it didn't, they would see me in a couple of weeks for the viability scan.

The bleeding did settle, and I carried on as normal as I could. I still worked, networked, went to the gym, and did my walks, and so on. The side effects of all the drugs had disappeared, and the main drug I was on was the vaginal pessaries to keep the womb lining thick and support the embryo to stay there.

I waited until week eight when it would be time for the viability scan, which would determine if it was again game over or if I would be transferred into maternity services and continue my journey to be a mum.

The day arrived, and again, my mum and I approached the hospital and waited patiently to be seen.

I went into the scan room, and the nurse asked how I was feeling. My reply was that I was nauseous as hell.

"Excellent," she replied. It was a really good sign I was beginning to feel nauseous, as it meant things were happening in the womb.

We did the transvaginal scan and saw for the first time the beginnings of the embryo and the life it was creating. The nurse asked if we wanted to hear the heartbeat. A big yes from my mother and me, and for the first time, we heard that tiny heart beating and alive. It was one of the most amazing and precious experiences for both my mum and me. We talked about it all the way home to my dad, and we told him about the awesomeness when we got home.

We knew we had a long journey ahead, but this little one was showing signs that it was here to stay with us for what was to come.

It was a bittersweet day as we were saying goodbye to the IVF department, which had looked after me for the last few years, and we were transferred into maternity services and a whole new adventure. It was a happy and sad day at the same time. I was sorry to be leaving the now-familiar IVF clinic, but I wanted to know what would happen and where my journey would take me.

I was permitted to stay at the hospital that I had all IVF with, so I was to move from the downstairs IVF clinic upstairs to maternity services and then, hopefully, ante-natal, labour and post-natal wards.

At this stage, there wasn't much else to do except wait and make friends with my community midwife, who would be supporting me through the next part of the journey.

# Part Two

# Chapter 31
## Pregnancy

I TOOK ONE day at a time with my pregnancy journey. I couldn't believe that I had been given the opportunity to go on such a journey, but I always knew that it could change at any minute. The last thing I wanted was to be filled with massive anxieties and have these override such a special time.

A pregnancy journey is a long, tiring, and emotional one at the best of times. Add into the equation that I was doing it solo, made it extra tiring and emotional.

But I wanted to do it, so I trusted my instincts and 'got on with it', which seems to be my nature.

My second and third in command started to take shape in the form of my parents. My mum would accompany me to the hospital appointments, and then my dad would be at home with cups of tea and be ready for that day's update.

I dealt with things when they happened, and I kept myself in as good a routine as possible the rest of the time. I went to the gym, ate as healthily as I could, kept working, and went to appointments when needed. Having a routine was a massive help to me during this time, as it was a distraction and a time to get things done.

Nothing changed in the first few weeks other than needing to pee a lot more and feeling tired, but then a lot of different things began to happen.

## Tiredness

Oh, that tired thing had a mind of its own. I would be in mid-conversation with someone and suddenly need a nap. I would fall asleep multiple times a day, especially when watching the telly.

Car trips as a passenger were a nightmare as you could guarantee I'd have a nap or two, even on a 20-minute journey.

I remember one occasion when I was on holiday with my family and fell asleep on my mother's shoulder in the middle of a tourist attraction. Apparently, a guide came to see if we were OK. My mother said something along the lines of everything being all good and explaining I was pregnant. The guide nodded and moved away to check on something far more cultural and job-worthy.

I also remember the ferry crossing from one of the Orkney Islands to mainland Scotland when all my family tried their best to keep me awake so that I would sleep on the crossing and try to avoid the sea sickness thing that was causing a bit of an issue. They tried and managed to succeed quite well, which meant I missed out a lot on the ferry back. I would always get a run-down of events when I woke up in case I missed anything crucial from the conversations I'd missed during nap time. I greatly appreciated this as I could keep going as best I could and felt included in everything that was going on around me.

At times, I had to watch what I did in the day and see how much energy I had used and how many minutes of naptime I could permit myself before moving on to another activity. I would have to plan my days in advance to allow me to work well, check in with whoever I needed to check in with, go to the supermarket, go to the gym if I had the energy and make sure the house was tidy.

If something was last minute and popped into the diary, the likelihood was that if it was urgent, it would be done, but if it wasn't, then it would be left. It meant I didn't get to go to a lot of evening events as I was usually fast asleep by eight or nine o'clock most nights.

I missed out on comedy shows, cinema, coffee evenings and music nights, but the end result was going to be worth it, and as a big advocate of listening to your body, I was doing just that.

I remember thinking about all the different places I'd fallen asleep, but the funniest time was on the concrete patio at my parents' house after a five-mile walk one sunny day. I woke up when a loud seagull flew overhead, and wondered what the earth had happened and why I was lying on concrete.

My mother confirmed I had indeed been asleep for around 20 minutes before she asked if I would like some juice to help wake me up a bit before I had to drive home.

People would try their best to keep me awake, but more often than not, it was a lost cause. My body needed sleep, and sleep was what it got.

The first trimester (1 to 12 weeks) and second trimester (13 to 27 weeks) were the worst when it came to sleep, but as I entered the third trimester (28 to 40 weeks), it did start to calm down and I could stay awake for longer. I would still go to bed early.

But there were days when I could skip a nap and be more present in the day and/or activity.

Again, it was all about planning and prioritising what needed to be done in the day or sometimes the whole weekend and being aware that if I had a busy day with work and a trip away from my home office across the country, then I would be paying for that the next day or the day after that.

## Nausea

Oh my goodness! I was one of those unfortunate women who ended up with nausea for eight of the nine months of my pregnancy. It was pretty annoying and seriously cramped my style in what I needed to do on a daily basis, with exercise, food and drink.

When the sickness first started, it was mild, but as the months progressed, the intensity increased. It appeared around the start of month two and set up camp. I remember thinking (and checking the internet) for when it should disappear. According to my research, morning sickness might start in the second month but usually disappears by month four or five.

I want to know who called it morning sickness because it most certainly was not just a morning thing for me. Every time my heart rate increased, the nausea increased, seriously affecting my exercise regime. Even mowing the lawn or walking upstairs started to be an issue. I had lots of nausea, but thankfully, I was only physically sick once.

Nausea is a strange thing as it can manifest in different ways:

- Feeling like your stomach is in your throat
- Getting that stingy, heartburn type
- Physically throwing up
- Feeling tired and drained
- Any movement, even just walking, can be a trigger
- Food and drink are no longer enjoyable
- Food or drink you tolerate one week, makes you nauseous the next week.
- Dehydration can result in a hospital trip
- You feel generally miserable and irritable

Of course, then there will be people who like to tell you their story and sometimes rub it in your face, saying things like,

"I didn't get sick."

"My pregnancy was a breeze."

"I wasn't sick once."

"Have you tried ginger, ginger ale, or lemon?"

I know these people were trying to help, but at the time, it was not useful.

Now, one of the weirdest things I had when I was nauseous was that I was unable to use my normal toothpaste and mouthwash. It was its minty strength, and unfortunately, it made me gag. That was not a good thing when you were trying to keep your teeth healthy and oral hygiene top-notch. I would try to brush my teeth once a day to keep them healthy, but after that, it was a bit of a lost cause.

I was in the supermarket one day during my prep for little one, and I looked at toothpaste and other things for children. I wondered if I could use them as an adult as they seemed lower in minty strength than the normal ones. I gave it a whirl, and it helped massively. I still gagged when brushing my teeth, but it was a lot better than the stronger stuff. Suddenly, my bathroom was home to kids' toothpaste and mouthwash. Again, if it worked and, bearing in mind it was only temporary, then that is what had to be done.

So, all in all, it was not a good place to hang out. At least I had an endpoint, which was some good news, but the days, weeks, and months on the road to the end point took time, effort and resilience on another level.

If I could sum up pregnancy nausea in two words:

It sucked!!!

## Chapter 32

## Through the Double Doors

THE SCAN APPOINTMENT waiting room at the hospital was next to some double doors that always intrigued me and my mum when we went for our appointments. We saw a lot of people and staff going through them and always wondered what was down that corridor. From the sign, it said acute medical wing, so we concluded it was a stopgap for things to be looked at before going up to the antenatal or labour wards, depending on what you presented with.

We both said it didn't look like a good place to hang out, as it meant that something was potentially wrong with the pregnancy and needed intervention, and made a pact to stay away from the double doors.

Well, that went swimmingly well until I was about halfway through my pregnancy, and my nausea ended up with nausea. My goodness, I woke up one morning feeling absolutely horrendous. It was summer, so I thought it was just the heat, but when I stopped eating and drinking, I knew something was very, very wrong.

Initially, I called my own GP surgery, who were worse than useless. I explained what stage of pregnancy I was at, the fact I had not eaten or drunk anything since the night before, and could I have an emergency appointment to see about some different medication to sort this out. The receptionist very curtly told me I was not deemed enough of an emergency to get an urgent appointment. I was left really not knowing what to do.

I called my own community midwife in floods of tears and, between crying, tried to explain what had happened and the fact I had called my own GP first. Her response was that I should have been taken more seriously but to call the pregnancy hotline at the hospital as soon as possible. I had to keep my own midwife posted, and I was to see her the next day for checks anyway.

I called the hospital and again told my story. Again, the nurse re-iterated that this was an emergency and I should have been dealt with by the GP as a matter of urgency with the stage of pregnancy I was at.

Needless to say, I was expected on arrival at those double doors for hospital checks, as this could have been dangerous for both little one and me.

The walk from the car park to the hospital was memorable for all the wrong reasons. Now, this walk for a normal person was about a medium-paced walk that would take around five minutes. Depending on where you parked, you went down a couple of flights of stairs, up one more flight, across the road, round the building, up another couple of flights or a hill, then you went down the stairs and finally into the building to go back upstairs either via flights of stairs or lift to the second floor.

Needless to say, I used the lifts where I could and was slower than a snail's pace on any stairs I had to use. The walk took around 15 to 20 minutes to get from the car park to the mini pregnancy A&E. Every time my heart rate went up when I walked I would have a hacking cough, which meant I had to stop to deal with it before continuing.

As I say a nightmare and memorable for all the wrong reasons.

A bundle of hospital tests ensued, and the conclusion was that I was dehydrated, needed stronger nausea meds, and I was to be kept in the hospital stop gap area for a few hours under observation before being sent home with a chaperone for further observation then to check in with my own midwife the next day. Any issues from there, I was to report back to the hospital pronto.

Although we did end up through the double doors, there was a highlight, and it was hearing little one's heartbeat loud and clear through the little monitor thing. They seemed to be doing fine in there, and it was just me feeling the effects of everything.

We came to the very firm conclusion, with my track record, that I tend to have a sensitivity to all hormones, and the sickness was part of it all. Lucky me!

It took around two days to get my hydration and food levels back where they should have been, but I got there in the end.

It was obvious the next day when I went for the midwife appointment how dehydrated I was as it took her three attempts to get blood out of me, and I was left with three gorgeous bruises to tell the tale. I was also told if there was to be a next time to bypass my own GP. A note would be put on my record that I must be seen at the hospital if anything else cropped up and needed attention. As my GP was worse than useless, I agreed that was a good way forward, and one that I could get on board with.

Now I say my GP was worse than useless, and I mean every word of it. It took several phone calls to get my nausea meds sorted, and every time my midwife sent down what I should be on, it was changed to something else. I had wee notes left on my prescriptions about what I should be on, I had phone messages left, and when I tried to return the call, no one would answer. The GP prescription line messed up what I had asked for, and everyone at that particular practice had absolutely no idea what to do with a pregnant lady with extreme nausea.

I remember one time I phoned in my script about a week in advance and deliberately took a screen print on my phone of when I had done it and when I went to pick it up. Apparently, they had no recollection of this. Well, that was until I showed them my screen print, and suddenly, within the hour, the script was waiting.

I had to stop my scripts from going from GP to pharmacy to keep a closer eye on everything, as the number of times things got lost on the way was not funny.

I don't know what it is about GP receptionists and where they managed to lose their customer service skills, but it was awful trying to get anything fixed. I was always second-guessed and made to feel like a criminal when I was just fighting for what was right for me.

I remember another particular time when I had to go into the surgery to see what had happened. I didn't raise my voice, but I admit I did have a slightly stern approach to the situation as it was once again the surgery that had messed up what I had asked them to do. Another receptionist suddenly appeared from around the corner to see what was going on, and I was made to feel like a thug demanding treatment. It was not a pleasant experience at all. I knew it was the GP at fault as, again, within a half hour this time, the problem was rectified.

As I like to say, customer service is a dying art these days, and in my opinion, everyone should be treated fairly and respectfully. Well, that's what all the posters in the surgery say anyway!

Another note to point out was that you could tell what stage of pregnancy I was at because of where we parked the car and who the designated driver was. We started in the car park, a 20-minute walk away, with me doing the driving, then we moved to the 10-minute one with me driving, and finally we moved to the five minute walk with my mum driving. I found it quite funny that you could tell what stage I was at just by the car parks.

# Chapter 33
## Pregnancy Nutrition

NOW MIGHT BE a good time for us to take a look at pregnancy nutrition.

As I have just said, with sickness, any nutrition was going to be tricky. In any pregnancy, there are dos and don'ts on what you are allowed to eat and, what you have to be careful of and what is a complete no, no.

Some of the elements were easy for me as I didn't have them in my diet at all. Things like alcohol and caffeine were easy to exclude. I occasionally had a fizzy pop, but not near the caffeine levels I had to avoid, so I was all good. Anyway, fizzy pop made the sickness worse, so I started to avoid it. Avoiding things like raw seafood and raw meat again was easy as yuck! Cheese and pâté were two other tricky ones that restricted my already limited cheese selection as

I couldn't eat unpasteurised cheeses. That meant I could only eat hard goat cheese and not much else. I occasionally eat pâté when I can find the right one without dairy or added gluten, but this was a no-go during pregnancy.

Then came weird things like avoiding pineapple and grapes. I'm not a massive grape fan, but I do like pineapple, so that meant no pineapple juice and no sticks of it, either. I can't remember the reasoning behind it all now, but they were to go on the no list.

The one thing that was difficult for me was tuna. Apparently, during pregnancy, you can only eat it twice a week because of its mercury content, but as it was one of the foods my stomach could handle, it was a bugger with the restriction.

One good thing, though, was eggs. As long as they were super-duper-cooked, I could eat as many as I wanted. They also agreed with me, so I had many different styles of eggs with toast, waffles, hash browns and baked beans.

I tried ginger ale, crystalised ginger, hot ginger tea, and anything ginger, but nothing worked. My nausea was to stay put despite my best efforts to get it under control with the help of food.

So, what could I eat? Well, it involved a diet of crisps, crisps, crisps and some more crisps. I found the vinegary crisps would calm the nausea for a few seconds. I could eat as many or as little as I wanted from the pack, and although not overly nutritious, it did seem to work. Apart from crisps, I ate watermelon, or any melon for that matter, sandwiches and pizza. The pizza thing was massively helpful when a new pizza takeaway place opened near where I lived, and I could pop down and order a pizza. Even better, it was all healthy for me because it was gluten, dairy and soya-free. I admit I had pizza multiple times in the week. Occasionally, I also had garlic bread, and what I didn't eat during dinner was usually lunch the next day.

The one thing I did find semi-useful was lemon sherbet sweets or lemon bonbons. I ate a bucket load until my local shop sold out, and I couldn't find them anywhere. A massive disaster as far as I was concerned, but in the middle of nowhere, after an overnight working away, I found both, and I stocked up. And I mean stocked up with around six bags of them!

I was waiting for that reported time during pregnancy when I could eat whatever I wanted and as much as I wanted, but it never came. All I could think of was that if all went well and little one was born in December, I could make up for eight months of a nauseous pregnancy diet by eating everything I could lay my hands on during December and into January.

To summarise, if I had one craving throughout pregnancy, it was probably for crisps and pizza. It was not highly nutritious or anything like that, but it kept me and little one doing what we needed to do.

I would say that so long as something is going into the tank to keep everyone doing what needs to be done, then go for it. You can always start the healthy eating thing on the other side of your journey.

As a side note, I was also lucky in the fact that I avoided any diabetes and glucose tests. Right at the start of the pregnancy, it was said that with my BMI and age, it was very likely that I would need to be tested for gestational diabetes, but when the time came, my midwife checked everything and ticked the box to say that I didn't have to go.

From what I am led to believe, the diabetes and glucose tests are four-hour tests with a glucose drink and blood tests, so a good morning or afternoon out of the day and with potential consequences and more drugs to take.

I admit that I felt very lucky that I could avoid all of this.

# Chapter 34

## Appointments, Scans and Injections

NOBODY TELLS YOU this, but believe me, being pregnant is a bit weird. There are a lot of appointments at the beginning of proceedings, then a long time in the middle where not much happens, before heading towards the 'big event' when the appointments increase again.

In a normal and healthy pregnancy, the appointments towards the end are not as frequent as I had, but with my IVF history, I was going to be kept a close eye on. I had no objection at all as I knew it was for the well-being and safety of us both. So, I turned up to every single appointment made for me.

The first appointment after I was discharged from the IVF clinic was with my community midwife, who was absolutely amazing. I couldn't have asked for anything more from her. She kept us updated as to when we needed to do things, explained what the process was, went through all the questions I had with great explanation and detail, and best of all, she made sure I understood everything I needed to. I was in charge of this operation, and my wishes were respected, which I loved.

My community midwife did things like blood pressure, taking blood for various tests, running through my birth plan (with plans A, B, C and the like), and answering any questions I had. She was also the person who gave me my flu jab, as they had one spare from the morning clinic when I was there. She even organised my COVID booster as well. It was great to be able to stay local for some of the many appointments throughout the pregnancy journey. As you can imagine, having gone through a lot of IVF appointments, I was a little tired of hospitals, so this was excellent for me.

The hospital appointments dealt with things like scans, a discussion with the anaesthetist about epidurals (or spinal injections), so we were prepared just in case we needed it, check-in with my consultant and further bloods. The hospital was also in charge of the 'big event', but more on that shortly.

The scans were absolutely amazing watching my tiny person grow month by month and develop. The first big scan at around 16 weeks was to tell us the sex of the upcoming new arrival. To be honest, I wasn't fussed either way as long as the baby was healthy. Just as everything else seemed to need repeating, so did the sex scan as little one had managed to get themselves cooried into the back of the womb at the top and turned towards my spine. No amount of jumping jacks, high knees, or thumping down on the scan table would move baby. Baby was snuggled in and staying put, so I ended up back in the scan suite the following week.

I had a feeling it would be a boy, but as it turned out, it was a girl. I remember saying,

"That's my daughter."

The scans after that monitored growth; I was scanned at weeks 28, 32 and an IVF special of 36. It was deemed she was doing well, and we would be welcoming her into the world within a matter of weeks. IVF folks get the extra scan as, any time from here, you may be looking at a quick trip to the maternity ward for induction. The reasoning behind this is once little one is 'cooked', they don't hang around and want them out. The longer little one stays in, the more risk there is of complications. As one doctor said to me, "You didn't do all the IVF hard work for there to be an issue now." It all made sense to me.

My thought was that it would be best to get the final prep done.

Other than the nausea taking me through the double doors at the hospital, there was one more noteworthy thing that happened, which was less than exciting. Blood thinning medication injections. Ouch! I was put on these due to my age and because I'd had complications through my IVF. The hospital also wanted to keep us both healthy. My goodness, those wee injections hurt like there was no tomorrow. The state of my stomach after those wee things was awful. I was black and blue, swollen, lumpy and sore. I had three months of them pre-birth, then a further three months post-birth. I had to get used to them, whether I liked them or not. I understand they were a necessary evil, but they were not fun at all.

# Chapter 35
## Memorable Moments

DURING MY PREGNANCY there were a few very memorable moments.

## Hearing a Heartbeat

I felt very fortunate when I was in the IVF clinic for the viability scan as I got to hear my little one's heartbeat loud and clear.

The next time was a few weeks later with my community midwife, and it was the most amazing sound in the world. My midwife even let me record it so I could listen to it at home. The recording sits on my phone to this day, and it is my most precious piece of audio. It brings a smile to my face whenever I hear it.

The following time, I was in the hospital through those double doors, and again, it was a very special thing to hear such a wonderful sound.

## First Kicks

One night, I fell asleep way before my phone clicked into its sleep routine thing. My phone goes on to 'do not disturb' and stops me from playing games late at night when the phone goes on to grayscale.

I was woken by the chime and got a fright, but so did little one, who seemed to go fluttering around the inside of my womb. It was adorable, and for the first time, I realised that we were both fully connected. When I got a fright and jumped, little one would also get a wee fright and did a jump, which I felt as a flutter in my stomach.

There were two other noteworthy times when I could feel my little one's movements that I still remember to this day.

The first proper kick was, unfortunately, to my bladder, and it was a tad on the ouchie side. I was driving up the motorway when it happened. It was lovely to feel little one move around in there, but at the time, I wished the baby could have picked a slightly less intense moment.

The second time, thankfully, I was on the train and not driving when the kicking happened, and I was able to enjoy it a bit more. Although it was slightly uncomfortable and made me jump, it was a lovely experience.

As the pregnancy developed, I could see my stomach moving when little one kicked. I tried to capture these moments, but I swear the baby could sense when my phone was out and waiting, and she stopped moving. Then, as soon as I put my phone away, the kicking started again. One afternoon, I was determined to film some action and over the course of an hour, managed to get a little tiny movement or two for my photo reel.

# Chapter 36
## Looking After My Back

I HAVE TO admit that I was actually very lucky with my back history and pregnancy. I did have an issue about halfway through, but with regard to severity, it was on the milder side.

It may have been all the mobility and work that I had been doing to keep my back as healthy as possible, but in terms of time, I think I was only sore and out of action for around ten days. Compared to my back injury in 2022, where it was four months, this was a good sign.

I think the other thing that helped was I noticed the signs very quickly and got help and interventions started as soon as possible.

I contacted the hospital physio department, and they had me in a pelvic pain clinic a few days later. I learnt so much in the 90-minute class that would help me massively going forward. Little things like having a pillow fort in your bed or wherever you were resting. I had about 15 pillows at one point to be comfortable. A pillow for my knees, one behind my back, one for my head, one for my feet, and a pillow for a pillow in case one of them got lonely. Times that by two as I had a bed and a couch, you can imagine how quickly these things grew. I went with the concept that if it helped, I was all for it.

The diagnosis of my back was that everything was relaxing with the hormones and my hips ending up out of alignment, which then ultimately pulled my back and aggravated my SI joint. Towards the end of the pregnancy, my calves got tired, and my hips ached, but with some light massage and stretching, I managed to keep them under control.

As I said, I was lucky that my back was only out for a matter of days, and I could take care of it at home with home remedies. I may have looked squint, but it managed to rectify itself as quickly as it had come on.

Other problems were that I struggled to reach forward on the rowing machine in the gym for the handle, my shoes seemed further and further away (slip-ons becoming the norm), and I had trouble moving with the bump.

Now let me tell you something here. There is a massive difference between social media pregnancy exercise and real life.

Do not believe everything you see!

If you are nine months pregnant and want to do high-intensity interval training with burpees and box jumps to post on social media and say, 'Look at me,' then go ahead.

But, and this is a big but, it isn't for everyone!

There, I said it, but now let me explain my reasoning. I always like to back my evidence with science.

If (and again, it is a big IF) you're having a healthy pregnancy, then go ahead with higher-intensity exercises. But, if you're having a pregnancy with complications, then you need to re-evaluate and do what is right for you and your baby.

Suppose you have back pain, hip pain and extreme nausea, which involves getting seriously sick as soon as your heart rate goes a millimetre above normal. In that case, burpees and box jumps are most definitely not for you, unless you want to cause some serious damage to yourself and potentially your little one.

I would always say even a little walk around the block at the slowest speed is better than nothing. I admit that even though sometimes that was a struggle for me, my life's motto of the healthier I am going into a situation, the healthier I will be, and the quicker I will recover led me slowly around the block, one foot after the other.

It all comes down to what you can do as a person and then as a person carrying and growing a smaller human inside you. The body goes through a lot during pregnancy, so the best words of advice I can give you is to listen to your body like it is your best friend in the world. Your body will soon tell you when it needs sleep, food, rest, a hug, a shoulder to lean on, someone to help you out, a day of smiles and sunshine, and everything in between. As long as you have good communication, your body will let you know what it needs, wants and would like.

However, sometimes, listening to your body can be tricky. We often hear what it is saying, but it tends to fall down in the action stages. When the body needs rest, it is best to let it do so, this way you don't end up with a knock-on effect and extreme fatigue, potentially becoming ill.

When I needed to pull back at the gym, rest a little longer in between what I was doing, or only do the bare minimum during my sessions, that was what my body needed.

I remember having to say goodbye to the adductors and abductors around the halfway point as there was too much pressure on my hips and pelvis, making things very uncomfortable. I stopped some of my ab work as there came a point where I couldn't lie on my back. I amended my weights to lower ones with higher reps and did what I could. If I went to the gym and did 30-60 minutes on the bike with a little bit of stretching thrown in, that was my workout for that day. At least I had made it. I did miss my box jumps and my high-intensity stuff, but I was carrying precious cargo, so I had to listen.

# Chapter 37
## What Shall I Buy?

I DIDN'T MAKE a lot of preparations for my baby until I was at the halfway point through the pregnancy and then again at the six-month point as well.

A friend gave me some excellent advice: to try charity shops for baby things, and she named a couple she thought would be helpful. This sounded like a perfect plan as I would save a small fortune and then be able to return the majority of the stuff to the shop for someone else to use or to sell it on and recoup some of my money.

Off I toddled one afternoon to one of my local charity shops in Bishopbriggs, which specialises in children's clothing, equipment, and toys.

All I can say is that I was like a deer caught in headlights. There was sooooo much stuff.

The thoughts that ran through my head were:

- Wow!
- What the heck do I need?
- How much do I need?
- Do I need to get that, and that, and that, or does that one do all three things?
- Do I get different sizes, or start with just one and build from there?

The list could go on.

I was very lucky that one of the shop assistants clearly saw the colour drain from me (not nausea this time!) and the look of bewilderment on my face because she came over and asked if I would like a tour and some advice. A big yes from me, and I was shown the baby equipment room, clothes, books, toys and bigger toys.

She explained clearly how everything came in, was sorted and then went out on to the shelf for purchase. I asked a couple of questions, and I left with some books, some clothes and a list of things to look further into.

I stayed true to my word (almost) for all the preparations, and most of my little one's things came from the charity shop, and I saved myself a small fortune along the way. I bought new car seats and mattresses for safety, a changing table and a cold-water steriliser.

The way I thought about it was one giant baby stuff library that you borrowed what you needed at that time, used it, and then, if it was still good, it went back for the next person.

So that was the 'stuff' preparations sorted, and I did it little by little so my bank account didn't get a fright and I wasn't going to get crazily overwhelmed. Over the months, I got everything I needed, researched a few bits for later on, and did what needed to get done.

I remember a couple of weeks before my little one was due, I had a flat full of tiny clothes on my drying rails. It was quite a sight. I then began to put some of the toys out and arranged for someone to come and help me put some stuff into the loft and make the changing table. Thank goodness for family to help me get the final prep ready.

I then got other bits ready for my parents' house and slowly moved in everything that we would need for the first few weeks of life. The plan was that close to the end of my pregnancy, I would move in with my parents and stay with them until into January, when I would hopefully be well enough to take us both safely back to my flat.

# Chapter 38
## Antenatal Classes

AS PART OF your pregnancy journey, you will probably be offered antenatal classes, where a midwife will go through your labour journey and explain what to expect, facts about breastfeeding, and the first few days with your new bundle of joy.

Now, a lot of the information was useful in these classes, but in the year 2023, I also thought a few things were lacking.

The first was that 'Dad' was used constantly when referring to the person going to be with you during labour, holding your hand and helping you with your first bathtime after the baby is born. It really narked me as I was definitely not going to have my baby's 'Dad' in the picture, and my mum was scheduled to be my birth partner.

As I say, in 2023, I would have thought this would be more on point.

In a room of 30 people, of which 15 were couples, how many were actually couples? Although it was mostly boy/girl, we could easily assume the fact, but in reality, what if we had three couples where the boy was a friend and the lady was doing the baby thing on their own, or their partner/husband/boyfriend worked away? What if we then had two lesbian couples who were going to be partners to go through it? I am sure you are beginning to see my point here.

At one meeting, I said, "Is it OK if the dad isn't in the scene as we are doing a generational thing, and my little one is going to have a single parent along with two incredible grandparents, and that was going to be my team?"

The midwife in question got a bit flustered and said something along the lines of, 'that would be fine'.

The second thing that annoyed me was the pressure and overload of information about breastfeeding. I know breast is best for little ones, but what if you get through to the other side having had a caesarean section where the milk doesn't come in right away, and the little one is starving? You are almost deemed a bad mother if you cannot breast feed.

I feel there should have been more reassurance and information about formula feeding in those antenatal sessions just in case your baby is formula-fed and not a breastfed baby.

And just while we are on the topic, many children have been formula-fed over the years and turned out OK.

I do wish more education had been used in the hospital, but hey ho, it was not to be, so I made it work with the best know-how I had, and I was more concerned about my baby going hungry rather than any social standard.

And there you have it.

Did I learn much from my antenatal classes? Not much, I'm afraid.

Did I learn heaps from my mum, the internet and from reading various books? Absolutely yes.

But I did learn of one way to get labour to start. Apparently, according to the midwife, you can start labour the same way the baby was made.

Sex!!!

That may be true in 'normal' circumstances where a nice Friday night, with a lovely meal may lead to one thing leading to another, but in my case, not so much.

My mum and I looked at each other after that was said, and giggled. There was no way, and I mean NO WAY, I would be getting little one out the same way she went in. I would just have to wait patiently until little one decided it was time to arrive safe and sound.

# Chapter 39

## Just a Routine Appointment

I HAD MOVED to my parent's house about a week before this particular appointment as I had been experiencing Braxton Hick contractions (which are a bit like labour contractions) and wanted to be somewhere where I had folks that could get me to the hospital if I needed to go in as soon as possible.

The Braxton Hicks didn't really amount to much except for being painful and uncomfortable. We called the hospital to make sure there was nothing we needed to do and were told to sit tight and that, unless they increased or a puddle appeared on the floor, there wasn't much to do.

My routine appointment on that Monday rolled around. We knew they would check on little one's heart rate, check my blood pressure and then do a vaginal sweep to see if there was any movement. We said goodbye to my dad before venturing to the hospital and sat perfectly happy in the waiting room chatting, admiring their Christmas decorations, discussing what was on the dinner menu back home and waiting our turn.

My turn came, and into the consulting room we went. First up was my blood pressure, and oh my goodness, it caused an issue. Three machines and four readings later, the nurse concurred that my blood pressure had spiked so much that the machine was having trouble reading it. It had been fine for the nine months previously, but that day, it had shot up.

Next came the vaginal sweep, where the nurse checked to see if the membrane could be separated from the amniotic sac. This, in turn, should release prostaglandins, which could start labour. Mine wasn't playing ball, and after the nurse, then the student nurse, and the nurse again had tried, it was deemed I could still be in for a wait, but the nurse would go and consult with a consultant who would have the final word on the next steps.

The next thing I knew, the consultant came into the room to chat. She explained that my blood pressure had probably spiked as there was a lot of pressure on my body, and I had started to get tired from all the hard work I had to do. As they already had me booked in for induction the following week, the consultant said that I was to go upstairs and, as long as my blood pressure settled, I would start the induction process that evening and that someone on the antenatal ward would come and speak to me about the plan. In short, she was saying that I was not leaving hospital without my little bundle of joy tightly wrapped in my arms.

Ooft! It was only meant to be a routine appointment.

The next thing I knew, I was wheel-chaired up to the antenatal ward. As my blood pressure had spiked, I was to be kept a very close eye on until it had come back down to normal, and that meant being wheeled around and not being allowed to walk anywhere.

So, off upstairs to the antenatal ward I went. Very luckily, I got a private room where my mum and I could collect our thoughts, update the immediate family, and calm down a bit about what was happening. I was very grateful for that side room.

As my blood pressure settled, the induction process started. It consisted of little one and me being hooked up to a heart rate monitor before some medication was sent up my vagina to my womb. The process was repeated every few hours to see if my waters broke or if my cervix opened up.

Apparently, not much would happen overnight, but it would be into the following day, or even the day after that, but I was in the right place, so all was OK.

My mum was dispatched to go and get my hospital bags and a good night's rest before she came back bright and early the next morning to sit with me and see what the day held.

Not much happened on that Tuesday except for some more waiting, but as we were more than used to it, we knew exactly what to do. At various intervals, I had my observations done. I went for lunch, listened to my little one's heart rate on the monitor, napped, chatted, read, watched telly on my phone, and the like.

During my induction process, they had my baby's heart rate monitor on my belly so I could both see the little wiggly pattern and hear it. I found it very soothing to hear it, and I admit I took a wee snooze with that as my backing track. I mean, when they hook you up to that machine for 30 to 40 minutes, you use the time wisely.

The contractions started to come thick and fast and were incredibly painful, but again, I knew I was in the right place, and I just had to let nature take its course. Around 24 hours after the initial induction process started, I was checked by the consultant again, and it became apparent that my cervix was just not playing the game we needed it to play.

I had some options to talk through with my family regarding the next steps, and the consultant would be back later that evening for an update. My options were to do the whole induction process again with a 24-hour break, but I would have to stay in the hospital. I could do a balloon thing (a catheter-like device that tries to get the cervix to open to aid labour and delivery), or I could opt for a C-section. Now, all along, I had said that I wasn't fussed about natural labour or a C-section as long as it was safe and healthy for us both. My conclusion was the C-section for several reasons. At any point, little one could get distressed, I was getting tired, I could have a further failed induction, which could end up in a section anyway, and as natural labour just wasn't working with my body, I was looking for Plan B.

So that was decided I was put on the emergency C-section list, but not as a real emergency, meaning I could wait my turn, which I was fine with.

Another night ensued. I was still checked every so often to make sure both of us were OK, and I was fasted from midnight with just a tiny cup of water at seven o'clock, ready for the following day. Fortunately, I wasn't overly hungry because of the nausea and pain. The only major change overnight was some super-duper painkillers, as those contractions were having a great party, and I was not enjoying it.

Luckily, the painkillers were sleep-making, and I got a couple of hours of much-needed kip.

# Chapter 40
## The Day I Will Never Forget

LUCKILY, WITH THE lack of induction drugs, my contractions had slowed down and, although still there, were much less intense, which was a relief. My super-duper painkillers could go back to regular ones, which was lucky as come mid-morning, I had to stop them so I was ready for theatre.

Again, the day was very similar to Tuesday, as in I napped, chatted, watched telly on my phone, and the like. However, this day was broken up with nurses, doctors, and anaesthetists coming to see us to double-check everything, make sure I knew what was happening, and sign all the forms that needed to be signed. Oh, and two men came to sort the lights in my room.

It was around three o'clock in the afternoon, and I was getting pretty tired and a little bored. I was ready to meet my little one but had to wait patiently (not something I am good at). I had just said to my mum that it was getting late in the day and did she think I would be put on the list for tomorrow. Suddenly, a nurse appeared at my door saying to get ready as one of the theatre nurses would be up in about 10 minutes to take us to theatre.

I cannot describe the emotions I felt at that point. It went from being calm and relaxed to let's go in a very short space of time, and my emotions had trouble keeping up.

It was the weirdest thing. The nurse came to my door, confirmed I was the correct person, and asked if I was ready to meet my little one. It was as if we were popping down to the local supermarket for a pint of milk. It was incredibly weird as I felt fine, and all I had ever known was going to theatre when you were poorly to get something fixed.

We were ushered down to the waiting room opposite the corridor to the theatre, and there we sat with my little monkey toy, which was going to be given to little one immediately after being born (well, at least put into baby's cot). A monkey, as I always knew she was going to be a cheeky wee monkey.

Then into theatre we went.

I had always been told that birth partners were not allowed into theatre whilst they were getting you set up and ready, but the theatre staff got my mum ready and sat her in my eyesight so I knew where she was all the time as they got me ready. A great relief, I have to admit and an added extra in the keeping things calm stakes.

There were lots of people in the room doing their thing and getting things prepared. I could see the cot where little one would be checked before coming to me, and there were lots of tubes, wires and bits of kit, all waiting to play their part. Everyone was lovely and stayed true to their word by explaining everything and keeping things as calm as possible.

I had opted for a spinal injection, which was administered and, again, an interesting feeling as you begin to lose the feeling in your legs. I had to admit that I felt absolutely nothing when it came to the main event itself. I was more aware of the people trying to put cannulas into my hands and arm as they were struggling to find a spot as I was so dehydrated, and there was a problem with the original one.

## And then my baby was here!

It was awesome, beautiful, amazing and surreal all at the same time. I saw her being held up and opening her little eyes before adjusting to the outside world, and it was a wonderful experience.

Now, I have to refer to my mum for the next part as I lost a lot more blood than was useful and blacked out for a few moments. While they were getting me fixed and awake again, little one was taken for checks, let out an almighty cry, then wrapped in blankets and given to my mum, her grandmother, for a well-deserved hug.

My mum brought her to my head, and we had a cheek-to-cheek hug until I was stable enough to hold her on my own. It was all a bit bizarre, and I was amazed that I had finally crossed the finish line.

Then, I finally answered the question of what her name was. I picked a name that was to be classic, Scottish, and to honour the donor's IVF initial when I decided which donor I would use.

Once I had been allowed off the theatre table and on to a proper bed (luckily using a slide board as I still had no feeling from my chest down), I had my own first hug with my new-born daughter, and it was extraordinary. After all the time, effort, complications, and heartache, I had completed the journey and could now hold my child. What a moment it was.

In case you were wondering, the reason my blood pressure had spiked was that little one had wriggled down (I told you she was wriggling before she knew what wriggling was, and she is still a wee wriggle monkey to this day) and was engaged, ready for delivery, but my body wouldn't let her out. Oops! The little red marks on her head attest to this and where she had been lying before being lifted out by the surgeon.

Also, everyone was correct; as soon as little one arrived and I had been sorted in theatre and on my way to recovery at some point along those lines, my nausea had finally disappeared, and it felt incredible.

I was wheeled into recovery and hooked up to an almighty bag of fluid to try and bring all my hydration levels back under control. I was also told to eat something to see if that would help the situation. And you never guess what! I was hungry, and I wasn't nauseous.

When we went into recovery, my mum started the ring round of our immediate family to say my little one was finally here. We even managed to sneak my dad into recovery for a quick hug with his new granddaughter. He had been patiently waiting at home for updates and the all-important news.

I was in recovery for a long while and began to think I would spend the night there, but finally, I was allowed to the post-natal ward for our first night as mother and child.

The recovery continued into the next day, and I felt the full force of what it felt like to have someone slice through my lower abdomen. I was shuffling, couldn't quite bend in the middle, and had my little one in tow wherever I went.

A lot went on in those days in the post-natal ward. As I had misbehaved during theatre with my blood loss and severe dehydration, I was kept under close supervision.

Little one also misbehaved and ended up in the neo-natal ward for a morning to be checked.

When babies are delivered naturally, they clear their little lungs on the way out, take their first breath, and live without any issues. In C-section, as they are coming out a different route, some babies do not clear their lungs, and it can lead to a chest infection, which needs monitoring. My little one did just that and ended up with a canula in her hand (and a massive board to stop her from pulling it out) and a course of antibiotics. However, saying this, I had my little one on my chest a lot for skin-to-skin and being close to mum, and after one round of antibiotics, she was deemed well enough. The doctor thinks she had been mimicking my breathing, and that is what helped and stopped her from needing anything further. She had her first x-ray at several hours old to check things were OK. She was also very jaundiced upon arrival and needed to be supervised for this as well.

Needless to say, we were kept in the right place for several days before we were finally allowed home to start our new life together as a family.

\*\*\*\*\*

Post-pregnancy, my back, hip and calf aches all disappeared, which was wonderful. However, I did end up almost immediately with swollen ankles and hives, which were seriously itchy, red and swollen. Luckily, it was only a few days of this before it disappeared. I mean, I shouldn't complain as I managed to get through all of the pregnancy with no swellings, so a few days of uncomfortableness was OK. I think this was due to the slow walking and slow biking in the gym just keeping the body moving.

I also managed to stand by my motto that I was healthy on the other side of pregnancy, and I did have a reasonably quick recovery. My main issues for not walking around my village was the weather. It makes sense when you have a little one at the end of November and into December, and the weather is notorious for being cold, icy, snowy and wet. To do what I could, when I could, was the easiest way, and I sat patiently waiting for a weather break.

# Part Three

# Chapter 41
## My Adorable Bundle of Joy

NOW, THIS ISN'T a parenting book in any way. It was never my intention to make it one. My journey is the story. However, there were a couple of little stories and information tips I couldn't leave out of the book.

One of the many first-day stories was when I asked my mum if my little bundle could be returned for a refund.

I had seen every hour of the clock as she cried. I tried feeding, white noise, music, dimmed lights, no lights, warm environment and everything in between, but still my little one cried. We ended up doing the thing that the midwives tell you not to do, and that was to fall asleep with me sat up and her lying on my chest. I think we got an hour or two that way as a last resort. Apparently, you can't return your bundle for a refund, so I was going to have to get used to 1, 2, 3, 4, 5, 6, 7, 8, 9, 10, 11 and 12 o'clock at both morning and evening time.

Thankfully, once we started to get into a bit of a routine in our new life, things settled down, and I began to see fewer of those times. I remember the first night I didn't see those early hours, and I woke with a start around five o'clock, wondering if little one was OK.

The second story that my mum tells is when the midwife came to do some checks on us. The midwife was wondering why little one was fast asleep in a baby bath with a duvet as a base and a blanket instead of in the baby box, which Scottish residents get and can be used as a bed. My mum answered,

"They have both had meltdowns, and I have just managed to get them both back down for a nap. Don't touch A-N-Y-T-H-I-N-G!!!"

We were, of course, both woken for checks, but my mum had good intentions.

The third story was after we had decided to stop breastfeeding around several days old. It wasn't working for both of us, and as a C-section, my milk didn't come in straight away and dried up. We both gave it a good shot, but it was not for us, and little one had to be formula-fed. The state of my t-shirts overnight with the hormone sweats and breast milk tidying was a sorry site. I was sodden each morning and required a change of t-shirt. I don't remember how many I went through in those early days.

Those are the main stories that stick in my mind. Of course, there are loads of others and many others to come too.

Regarding information and tips with a newborn, my main one is to listen and watch the baby. They soon tell you if they are hungry, need a hug, need a nappy change, just want to be close to you, or are sleepy. There is so much information about how to do things correctly and the best way forward, but reading your own child is the best way I know.

That also applies when something doesn't sit right with you; you don't need to do it. If social media says it is the bees' knees and you must try it today, by all means, give it a whirl, but if it isn't right or you don't like it, it doesn't necessarily mean you need to continue with it. Or that you are wrong or have failed.

Only you know what you have been through on the quest to have a child, which is your story and your story alone.

# Chapter 42
## One Final Thought

THERE IS NOTHING better after such a long and complicated journey than finally holding your adorable bundle close to you, for them to start to recognise you as their mother, and for you to recognise them as your child.

A few chapters ago, I wrote about whether I would do another round of IVF. I am very aware my IVF journey, although difficult, did have the most unbelievable result and one that I am very happy with. I have thought about whether I would do it again, but the short answer is no.

As much as I would love another child so that my little one has a little brother or sister, realistically, my body is not going to take another round of IVF, hormones, drugs, medical procedures and everything else. As I said during my second round, I was very close to an ICU admission, and my worst-case scenario is that my child might be left without a parent. So, considering all this, my answer to having another is a sad but understanding no.

Someone also asked me recently if, having known everything I went through on my IVF journey, I would have still gone through with it, and the short answer is yes, I would. I needed to be a mother with my egg, and I had to try, so yes, I would have.

I do believe there will be children in my future. I just don't know how they will all fit in yet.

I'm pleased to say that at the time of writing this book in 2024, it has become more common to have these elements heard and, more importantly, understood by people.

I think one of the next stages is to let single women access IVF through NHS, as that is a hotly debated topic. It is also a massive factor as to the reason why I have chosen to document my journey.

My hope is that one day, it becomes even more normal to hear these words.

# Acknowledgements

Thank you to my wee cheeky monkey (E) because without you, there would be no book.

Throughout the writing of this book, a few people have helped me along the way, and I would like to thank them.

Firstly, my family members, who have been on the entire journey with me and helped me through everything.

Secondly, my business mentor, who one day told me to finish the book and get it published.

Thirdly, my friends, who were always there with many a hot chocolate and walk.

Thank you to my proofreaders and helpers for believing that there was 'something' there to publish.

And to everyone else over the years who threw their two pence into the drama to see if it would help, an enormous thank you.

Lastly, you, my readers. Without you, there would be no need for a book.

# About The Author

You've probably got to know me a fair bit through this book, and as you can see, I have a big passion for walking, going to the gym, dancing, and, of course, hanging out with my little one.

You are always welcome to contact me about IVF, weight loss, nutrition and fitness.

I don't know all the answers, but even if you just need a rant after a bad appointment, I am always open to a hot chocolate in a cafe.

You can find me at:

HCActiveWomanFitness@hotmail.com

Insta/Facebook – HC Active Woman Fitness

# References

## NHS BMI Website

Calculate your body mass index (BMI) for adults - NHS (www.nhs.uk)

## BBC News on Gluten-Free

Is going gluten-free good for you? - BBC Food

## No Gluten Benefits

10 Benefits of Eating Gluten-Free - No Gluten

## Holland and Barrett

Going Dairy Free | Tips & Intolerances | Holland & Barrett (hollandandbarrett.com)

## NHS Foods to Avoid During Pregnancy

Foods to avoid in pregnancy - NHS (www.nhs.uk)

# Glossary of Terms Used

## CMV (Cytomegalovirus)
A common viral infection.

## Duathlon
An event in which you run, bike, and run, whereas a triathlon is a swim, bike, and run.

## Folic Acid
Is needed before and during pregnancy as it helps red blood cell development and cell function and is known to reduce the risk of Spina Bifida.

## IUI (Intrauterine insemination)
Fertility treatment where the sperm goes directly to the woman's womb during ovulation.

## IVF (In vitro fertilisation)
A type of assisted reproductive technology.

## Transvaginal Scan
Where a probe is inserted via the vagina to see the inside of the womb and ovaries.